MY SEVEN- DAY MAKEOVER

One Breast Cancer Survivor's Spiritual Journey

CYNTHIA W. TURNER

My Seven-Day Makeover

This book is dedicated to the men who
have most influenced my life.

To my husband, Kevin.

To my sons, Julien and Justen.

To my father, Rev. Franklin R. Williams.

To my brother, Clinton Williams.

In memory of my grandfather, the late Samuel W. Pinner.

Acknowledgments

———————— ❧ ————————

I give all honor and praise to my Lord and Savior, Jesus Christ, who gave His life so that I may live. I pray that I represented You well in this journey, and that this work is pleasing to You.

I thank my family, Kevin, Julien, and Justen for walking with me through this valley. Your love, strength, and laughter carried me during my weakest moments. I love you.

I thank my parents, Franklin & Mary Williams; my siblings (and spouses), Celia (Thad) Hopkins, Frances Williams, and Clinton (Kim) Williams; my grandmother, Hannah Pinner; my stepdaughter, Kia; and all of my aunts, uncles, cousins and in-laws for your love, support and presence. It really mattered.

I thank all of my many angels on this journey, including Susan Sutherland, Joella Jones, Dr. Charles Washington, Sr., Dr. Charles "Dari" Washington, Jr., and Christina Walker. You made my journey much easier. Thank you.

I thank all of my prayer sisters (and brothers) for your "knee duty" during my season of need. You were truly my lifeline. I am indebted to you.

I thank my extended family, members of CT & Heartspeak; my church family, Canaan Missionary Baptist Church; and my colleagues at the University of Illinois for your love and support. You are the best.

Preface

I was diagnosed with breast cancer on October 16, 2006. And to be perfectly honest, this news literally shook me to the core. I felt as if I had been emotionally blindsided and spiritually assaulted. For weeks, I could not wrap my mind around the thought of what this might mean. I could not begin to consider what it may suggest.

Was I scared? Unequivocally, yes! Cancer?! Come on. I was only 38 years old. I had a husband and two young sons whom I loved with every cell of my being. I had a fulfilling job and career. I had a growing professional music ministry. I was extremely active in my local church and loved serving my Lord and Savior, Jesus Christ. All I knew about cancer at that point was that it was a formidable opponent whose blow often could be quick and fatal; and if the cancer did not deliver the fatal blow, the treatments and their effects could be equally debilitating.

However, unlike what some would imagine, "why me?" was not my first question of interest. In fact, looking back, I am surprised that I never felt compelled to ask this. Perhaps, I had remembered from past difficult experiences how this question would often take me down this emotionally descending and spiraling path where I would revisit every one of my former acts of poor judgment and recklessness. Such a reflection often conjured feelings of worthlessness and futility. Or, maybe I had recalled from other challenging episodes how this question would frequently move me to compare my life and circumstances to those of others. This analysis would arouse, in many instances, emotions of injustice and self-pity.

Possibly, it was the enormity of the event that I was facing. I just could not fathom that it was solely for and/or about me. Thus, for whatever reason, on this occasion, I chose not to entertain the question of "why?" Instead, I asked, "What?" Specifically, I asked, "What is the purpose of this, Lord?"

Upon reflection, I praise God for this change in course of inward dialogue. The question of "what?" opened the door for me to hear God afresh. While the question of "why?" always led me to ponder the possible "because" answers with its focus solely on me and that around me, the question of "what?" allowed me to totally attune to Him, for only God in His sole omniscience could respond. As I sought to hear His discourse, the same scriptures I had read time and time before now took on new significance and meaning. The songs He had written on my heart in the past now spoke to a new audience of one—me. Prior challenges now seemed like pre-game activities in relation to this new circumstance. Most importantly, God revealed His answers to me in the context of the most well-known of scriptures, in the simplest of tasks, through the most unlikeliest of people, and with a sense of humor that unarmed my deepest worries and fears. Indeed, He took my physical battle and made it a spiritual classroom.

On the following pages, I attempt to share with you some of the insights from this journey. Included you will find excerpts from email messages sent to my prayer circle of Christian sisters who laughed, cried, and prayed with me throughout my healing process. I sincerely hope that my sharing of this journey will bless you as much as my experience of this journey has stretched me (which is a WHOLE lot).

Table of Contents

CHAPTER 1

"And we know that all things work together for good to them that love God, to them who are the called according to His purpose."
(Romans 8:28)

God employs all things to work in our favor so that we may be shaped in His.

From: Cynthia
Sent: Tue 10/17/2006 4:22 PM
To: Prayer Sisters
Subject: Prayer Warriors Needed

Hey, good folks. I just wanted to share with you a recent test that I have been given to enrich my test-imony. I have been diagnosed with breast cancer. (You know, just to articulate this is still so surreal to me.) I found out yesterday. The doctors believe that I am in the early stages, but I won't know for certain until after surgery. It is in my left breast and it is quite small at the moment (1.6 cm). Anyhow, I do have a peace about this because I KNOW that God is a healer. (Plus, there is still so much I want to do for Him—I know it is not my time *smile.*) I am asking for your prayers. Specifically, I am asking that you pray the following:

1) The cancer has and will not spread anywhere else in my body beyond that 1.6 cm nodule before they are able to remove it.
2) I continue to maintain a peace of mind about this.
3) Kevin will maintain a peace of mind about this.
4) I can endure whatever procedures that are required (even if I have to put my vanity in check and lose my hair- LOL).
5) My boys are not ill-affected by this process (I choose not to share much with them until it is clearly necessary).
6) I become the better and stronger physically, spiritually, and emotionally for going through it.
7) And foremost, God gets the total glory and victory!

I go to see my specialists next week and the procedures will be decided at that point. I will keep you posted.

Thank you in advance for your love and prayers.

Love y'all,
Cynthia

P.S. By the way, you do know that God knows how to balance things out, don't you? It was announced today that Kevin's current cd project of hymns entitled, "HIM," was formally nominated for the Stellar Awards 2007 "Instrumental CD of the Year." The event is January 13, 2007. So add just a slight addition to the prayer list, if you don't mind, that I will be healthy (and cute) enough to strut down the aisles of Grand Ole Opry in Nashville to be by my man's side at this event. (*smile*)

I have finally embraced the reality that, in this life, the unexpected will happen. In particular, I have come to terms with the certainty that we all will encounter in our lifetime our share of the unforeseen, the unannounced, and the uninvited. Really, I don't know why I have grappled with this matter for so long. The Bible clearly articulates that discord is the direct consequence of Adam's fall. Hence, I have always intellectualized this truth to be spiritually apparent. Nonetheless, I guess I have never accepted it to be person-ally applicable. To be honest, I think *what had happened was* that I had somehow tried to disown Adam in my genealogy. Ha! I just never could understand why Adam could not have resisted Eve regarding that darn tree. Life would be so much easier. Wishful thinking, I suppose.

Anyhow, it is now clear to me that all of us are suscepti-ble to life's travails. Moreover, difficulties can and will often come as a result of no fault of our own. Jesus spoke to this point in John 9:1-3 when asked about the cause of one man's blindness, "Neither hath this man sinned, nor his parents."

Consequently, no amount of money, education, or spiritual-ity exempts us from trials. (Let me say, though, that I believe that not all adversity is created equally. Some "drama" I suggest, we create ourselves.) Yet, to the extent that life's dilemmas are not self-evoked, I have concluded that there are no discriminatory practices involved in how they are distributed.

I praise God, however, that where our understanding ends, God's revelation begins. Thus, as I came to these sobering conclusions at the outset of one of my most challenging journeys ever, God began a dialogue with me that changed my life forever. He immediately showed me that these truths were not the final summation for the believer. Still, my acceptance of the carnal realities of this world was a necessary first in order for me to experience the spiritual provisions of His world. In essence, I had to be freed of my "trial denial" condition in order to take hold of God's "trial survival" provision, "…that all things work together for good to them that love God" (Romans 8:28).

I knew then, though, that God's discourse was not going to make for easy listening during my present trek. I already had a problem with His provisional inclusion of the term "good." You know why? Well, when I simply looked beyond my particular circumstance, for the life of me, I could not apprehend how the devastating and despondent events about which I daily read could be for our "good." Beyond my personal obstacle, I could not reconcile how the unjust and wicked actions of some against innocent others could be for our "good." Beyond my current predicament, I could not settle how the crippling conditions of the vulnerable and the horrific suffering of the oppressed could be for our "good."

However, God quickly reminded me that my issues were not novel. These age-old questions had been posed and pondered throughout the annals of time by both believers and nonbelievers. Further, many of these circumstances are simply artifacts of a secular world where free will exists. Yet, His stance has remained the same. God prompted me to again revisit His promise: "And we know that all things work together for good to them that love God, to them who are the called according to His purpose."

As I read this scripture again for the umpteenth time in my life, God brought back to my remembrance something my current pastor (B.J. Tatum) once shared with our congregation regarding this matter. He stated that God did not promise the believer that all things would be good. Instead, God promised that He would take all things (both good and bad) and work them for our good. That is, while all circumstances are not favorable, God employs all circumstances to work in our favor.

God then impressed upon me to go back to the first time He spoke of "good" in the scriptures (as if He could read my still-conflicted mind). And guess where I ended? At the beginning. That's right. He took me back to... the Creation. He took me back to a time where the scriptures say that in everything that He saw, "it was good." And, yes, He took me right back to that Adam dude who I had problems with in the first place! Ha! Moreover, for six months, God walked with me through my valley experience illuminating at each turn His original road map for that which He designed as "good" in the Creation. Further, as I traversed through my valley's rough terrain, God faithfully reminded me of the all-sufficient revision that He made to His road map to compensate for the first man, Adam, and his failed pursuit of "good." He faithfully reminded me of Jesus, the second Adam, who made it possible for all of us to experience "good" in its fullness. In turn, I soon discovered what God has always purposed "good" to be for man: "And God said, Let us make man in our image, after our likeness..."(Genesis 1:26). That is, God's definition of "good" for every believer is that our lives resemble His likeness.

So let me share with you how this image-enhancing journey began for me.

CHAPTER 2

"In the beginning God created the heaven and the earth. And the earth was without form, and void; and darkness was upon the face of the deep. And the Spirit of God moved upon the face of waters." Genesis 1:1-2

When in the dark about a situation, know that God is not. His movements you just can't see.

From: Cynthia
Sent: Wed 10/25/2006 9:56 PM
To: Prayer Sisters
Subject: For we wrestle not against flesh and blood...(ROUND 1)

Hey my praying sisters,

I'm going to try to make this short this go around. I met with the doctors yesterday. My day of surgery is planned for Monday, Nov. 20. They will do a lumpectomy (removal of the tumor) in my left breast and a sentinel lymph node dissection (the removal of several of my lymph nodes under my arm). This surgery will allow the pathologists to accurately determine the aggressiveness of my cancer, the stage of my cancer, and whether it has spread beyond my breast tissue. What I do know at this point is that my cancer is invasive (it has spread to the surrounding tissue), however, the tumor itself is smaller than I originally thought- at its maximum dimension, it is 1 cm. Thus, I am blessed that my doctor did find such a small spot. My next prayer requests of you are the following:

1) The cancer remains contained in the tumor and does not spread beyond the current affected breast tissue until it can be removed in surgery.
2) The lymph node results will come back negative of any cancer (this determines whether the cancer has likely spread).
3) The doctors will accurately assess my pathology report from the surgery and we will determine the treatment that will CURE my cancer.
4) I will experience no ill side effects from surgery.
5) My family and I will remain at peace throughout this process.
6) My boys will not be ill-affected through this process.
7) I will receive the best doctor care on this side of Jordan.

And, of course, please include that should God want to work a miracle (without medical intervention) at any time, HAVE AT IT! (*smile*)

You will be amazed how God is already transforming things in my life. I've already TOTALLY altered my eating (I will share more with you later about this). And, oh yeah, pray that God will cover our finances throughout this process. Eating healthy COSTS! I am already, though, seeing results of my change in diet.

Thanks so much for your incredible and continuous show of love and support. I love y'all! Your love reminds me everyday of the all-encompassing love of God. This is but ROUND ONE... (I'm sorry. I was trying to make this short.)

-Cynthia

From: Susan
Sent: Thu 10/26/2006 1:12 PM
To: Cynthia; Prayer Sisters
Subject: RE: For we wrestle not against flesh and blood... (ROUND 1)

Most Gracious, Heavenly Father, I lift up Cynthia to You at this very moment and thank you God for her complete and total healing in Jesus Christ's name!

I thank you God for the cancer to be non-existent in her body and in her life.

I thank you for no need of results of any kind since the cancer has completely vanished!

I thank you and lift Cynthia's doctors up to you Father, for the miraculous event they will witness first hand - with Cynthia's complete and total healing!!

I thank you God for Cynthia's continued good health and her feeling empowered, uplifted and the best she has ever felt!!!

I thank you God for her husband and her children, for their peace and believing at this time. For the prayers being lifted up to you and said on behalf of Cynthia and her loved ones.

I thank you so much Father, that we, her sisters in Christ, continue to stand and pray for her good health and, again, the witnessing of her healing.

I especially thank you, Most Gracious and Heavenly Father, for what your son, Christ-Jesus accomplished on that cross for Cynthia ...

In Jesus Christ's Glorious Name – AMEN!

---

*H*ave you ever looked back on particular circumstances in your past and realized later that God was simply setting the stage for your present? Let me further clarify. Think of a time when you were going through a situation and you had no clue why ("and darkness was upon the face of the deep..."). Now reflect. Looking at where you are today, could it be that back then it was "the Spirit of God moving upon the face of (your) waters?" Hey, hey, hey! Well, wait until I tell you about the behind-the-scenes events that led to the powerful email prayer response above!

But let me not move too fast. Of course, we all know that the providence of God (God's preserving, sustaining, ordering, ruling, and governing of His creation) flies in direct opposition to worldly notions of coincidence, accident, chance, luck and fortune, right? In fact, for the believer,

Psalm 37:23 says that, "the steps of a good man are ordered by the Lord..." So, in essence, as I have heard a-many-a preachers state, circumstances in which we find ourselves are either God-allowed or God-arranged.

I sometimes wonder, though, if we fully comprehend this point. For example, consider the term, "coincidence." Many folks often use this term to speak of event occurrences that they believe to be accidental or pure luck. What most don't know is that "coincide," the root form of coincidence, is a mathematical term which means to "correspond exactly" or "perfectly align." Question: Since when did accidents become part of an exact science, or luck a perfect calculation?

At least for me, I now recognize that I have often been so distracted by the sheer "busy-ness" of everyday life, that I failed to sometimes see how and when God was quietly and strategically shifting things around in my life—placing new people in, moving old ones out, shedding old habits, igniting new passions, etc. Of course, certain things such as the overtly obvious material blessings—a new house, a new car, a promotion, etc.—those have always been easy for most of us to attribute to God. But, lately I have taken the time to thank God for small things like prompting my sons to interrupt me (on more than one occasion) just right at the moment when I was about to put my foot deep in my mouth (*smile*). On a deeper level, I've started praising Him more for character improvements—letting go of negative emotions such as anger, worry, and fear more quickly (they are paralyzing); learning how to say, "I'm sorry" more readily (it's freeing); and not having to be the one that is right ALL the time (still working on that one, but getting better!). Well, one of the many praise offerings that I sent up was regarding a simple office move that took place right before my darkest night to date. Read on.

April 2006

Late one afternoon in April of 2006, I vividly remember receiving a phone call from Jean, my department administrator. She asked me would I be interested in moving to another office. Now, mind you, I had been in the same office since I first began at the university which had been close to eleven years then. Further, being the creature of habit that I am, I probably would have stayed there until I retired.

Have you ever met folks like this? (If my car bag phone had not died years ago, I would likely have been the only person on this earth still using one. Seriously! I am the epitome of what advertisers call a "brand loyalist." Once I get used to one thing, I stick with it— just because.)

At any rate, as soon as she began sharing with me about the possible change, all I could think about was moving eleven years of accumulated STUFF. And as if she knew what was going through my head, Jean immediately interjected all of the positive points. I would have at my disposal student office workers who would assist me in whatever way I needed in my packing and moving (okay...). I would get new office furniture (nice...). My new office had a window that had a better view than what I currently had (I can work with that...). Lastly, the new office location was situated in a bigger office space that was managed by a young woman named Susan, who was one of the department's secretaries. Jean indicated that should I choose to move, Susan could assist me in my current student advising duties (JACKPOT!).

The move took place that June, and it went as seamlessly as I could have asked or desired. After throwing away nearly half of the (unnecessary) items that were in my former office, sure enough, everything was in place and in order practically overnight. (I work for some of the best folks. Really!) A few days after the move, I formally introduced myself to Susan and told her that I looked forward to working with her. I was then quickly corrected.

"What do you mean?" I recall her asking. "I have not been told of a new work assignment. I am already working for two people."

"Oh. It was my understanding that you would be assisting me with my student advising schedule," I replied.

"Who told you that?" she asked.

By now, I was thinking, "Okay, let me stop while I am ahead. Maybe I hadn't heard Jean correctly." So I responded, "I'm sorry. Maybe I got it wrong," and quickly went to my office.

Once I closed my door, I immediately began a quiet rant of my own. "Lord, for eleven years I did fine in an office space all alone, not bothering anyone. I didn't ask for this move, and I definitely did not want to start things this way. Is this going to work? Or, should I ask for my office back before it's too late?"

No answer, of course. Ha!

Well, the next morning I felt a bit better. Before going into the office, I had decided that I would simply continue to be responsible for my student advising schedule. I just needed to work out logistics with Susan because the students would now have to walk through her office to get to mine, and I wanted to make certain that I was sensitive to how she wanted this handled.

When I arrived at the office, I promptly met with Susan and again reiterated my apologies to her regarding my presumption that she would be working with me. She responded that having just talked with Jean, she had determined that she would be assisting me. We simply needed to work out the details. (Look at God!) Consequently, we spent some time discussing my needs and agreed that she could best help me by handling my calendar. Little did we know, however, that something was about to take place that would alter our understanding of this arrangement forever.

September 27, 2006

It was the last Wednesday of September. I was due for my annual physical check-up. I had my to-do list prepared, and was anxious that afternoon to share with my doctor the procedures I wanted done over the next year. I had decided to once and for all take control of my physical health, and there were two procedures that were of utmost importance to me.

The first was a corrective foot procedure (women, read between the lines). It was at the top of my to-do list. You see, twenty years of walking in three and a half inch heels everyday had finally taken its toll.

In college, I can remember my girlfriends often asking me how I was able to walk across campus daily in heels. I suppose, you can call it woman's vanity. Heels were such a part of my college persona that when I would decide to wear tennis shoes or flats on occasion, my male friends would make it a point to tell me that I didn't look right in them.

Anyhow, the heels started causing me physical trouble after the birth of my second son, Justen. Similar to my first pregnancy, I gained a whopping 60 pounds on my 5' 3-¾" frame when carrying Justen, and my feet ballooned in the process. Still, I insisted on wearing the pointy toe heels and boots. I had to maintain my "cuteness" status quo, you know. Before long, though, I began intermittently experiencing a throbbing on the left side of my right foot. And after several years of ignoring it (self-imposed trouble written all over it), the problem became visibly apparent. I could no longer hide from my reality.

Second on my to-do list was fixing that hernia of mine. Again, this resulted after my pregnancy with baby number two, Justen.

Well, on the day of my appointment, I was just chatting away with my doctor regarding this wish list of mine as she was performing my chest examination. In the midst of our dialogue, she momentarily paused and then started prodding deeper under my left arm in one lone area.

"What's that?" I remember her asking.

"What's what?" I replied. (Writing is so therapeutic. Boy, was I in the dark during this period in my life.)

"Feel this." She tugged at the skin under my arm. I placed my fingers where hers had been and felt nothing unusual. It simply felt like she was pushing against my ribs.

"I don't feel anything."

She then pulled the skin tissue of concern away from my chest cavity and had me knead it with my fingers. As uncomfortable as this pulling and tugging was, I now felt what she was referring to. While it was extremely tiny and circular in shape, the lump was quite hard and grainy in texture; thus, the reason for why I thought that it was part of my rib cage.

"Okay, what is that?" I asked.

"Well, I am not sure," she answered. "It is most likely a fibro adenoma, a benign tumor that is quite common among African American females your age. But just to make certain, let's get it checked out."

October 16, 2006

The day of reckoning had arrived. I had undergone both a mammogram and ultrasound over the last two weeks, and the results were in. I fully expected the doctor to indicate that the spot noted during my annual checkup was benign. I was so confident of this that, weeks before, I told my husband Kevin that he needed not come to the follow-up appointment. I was certain that I would be in and out in no time. Naturally, he wouldn't hear this, so he said that he was planning on being there. But we both knew that meant I needed to remind him. You see, beside the word "forgetful" in the Turner's dictionary is a picture pasted of my husband!

I arrived at the clinic at about 2:10pm for my 2:00 o'clock appointment. (Me and time—another thing I am really working on!) I went through the normal check-in routine, and soon found myself in the doctor's office twiddling my thumbs.

Fifteen minutes went by. No doctor and no Kevin. Hmm. Another ten minutes went by; and again, no doctor and no Kevin.

"Okay, now what's going on?" I thought to myself. "And where in the heck is Kevin? He said that he was coming." Anxiety building, I tried ringing his cell phone, but couldn't reach him.

"Miss Invincible, you purposely didn't remind him of your appointment today, remember? You didn't think it was necessary for him to come. You know where he is. He's at work." I checked my voicemail to make certain that, by chance, I had not missed his call. Nope, I hadn't.

My confidence was now wavering a bit. I just could not understand why the doctor would leave me here to wait so long for results of this nature. After thirty minutes of sitting, I peeked outside the door, and inquired of one of the nurses walking by as to where the doctor might be. The nurse indicated that my doctor was running late, but was on her way to my room next.

"Calm down, Cynthia," I began to tell myself, "everything is going to be okay."

Sure enough, moments later, my doctor quickly entered the room. However, unlike her usual manner, she failed to look at me and offer some quick-witted comment about seeing me again so soon. Instead, she took her seat, opened her laptop, and commenced to read intensely that which was on the screen before her.

"This is not what I expected," she expressed grimly, her attention still directed toward the computer screen.

Ah-oh!

"What do you mean?"

She then turned and looked at me for the first time, "Cynthia, you have breast cancer."

She hesitated as if to give me a chance to absorb her statement, and then continued, "It seems to be quite small, and so we think we have caught it in its early stages…"

I remember interrupting her with a nervous laugh, "Oh, you are joking, right?"

"I wouldn't joke about a matter of this nature," she replied.

"Why can't I reach Kevin?!" I uttered fretfully under my breath while fumbling over the keypad of the phone to dial his number again.

She followed, "I need to set up appointments for you to meet with an oncologist and surgeon. Why don't I leave you alone to make your phone calls while I go and make your appointments. I'll be back shortly…Cynthia, I'm so sorry."

And suddenly I was left in the office by myself. Again.

Now, what on earth was I supposed to do?

I considered my alternatives at that point. Well, I could just fall out on the floor and sob uncontrollably, but then, no one would be there to console me. Ha! I could call Kevin and fuss at him for not being there, but number one, I can't get through, and number two, I was supposed to remind him of the appointment in the first place. Furthermore, this alternative really would be a displacement of my highly volatile emotions on to Kevin. Not fair and not mature.

Okay, what other alternative did I have?...

Aha! Call my mom and my dad!

"Hey dad," I said after my father picked up on the other end.

"Hey, Cindy! How are you doing?" he responded with his usual jolly self.

"Uh, not so good. The doctor just shared with me the results from my chest ultrasound."

"Huh? Well, look, here's your mom," he quickly answered, concern emanating from his voice, "Mary, pick up the phone, it's Cindy!"

"Cindy, hey. What's going on?" my mom asked as she got on the phone.

"Mom, I have breast cancer."

"What?" she quietly exclaimed.

I could tell that she was trying to stay calm; but that didn't last long. Shortly thereafter, she began rattling off fifty thousand questions, "What does that mean? Where are you? How are you? Where is Kevin? Where are the boys? Did you just find out? What's next?... " By that time, Kevin called. I told my mother to hold on for a second and switched over to the other line.

"Kevin, I am at the doctor's office. Please come."

"Oh! On my way."

I could tell from the tone in his voice I needed to say no more. Returning to my mom's conversation, I told her that I had shared with her all that I knew, and that Kevin was on his way. My dad got back on the phone and told me that he loved me and then prayed with me. I assured them that I would call as soon as I got further information.

Kevin rushed into the doctor's office with a knowing look on his face. He hugged me as the doctor returned to the room. The doctor then restated the facts to Kevin and indicated that I was to next meet with the oncologist (a doctor who specializes in the treatment of cancer). The oncologist would devise my treatment plan. My doctor suspected that my treatment would include a lumpectomy (the surgical removal of the lump), followed by either radiation alone, or a combination of chemotherapy and radiation. She further speculated that being that I was so young, my oncologist would likely pursue an aggressive treatment to ensure the best outcome.

As my doctor began providing me with the dates and times of my upcoming appointments, I suddenly heard faint, incoherent noises to the side of me where Kevin was sitting. I looked over, and guess what? My husband was quietly sobbing away! (You know the kind of sobbing where your face is all contorted, you mouth is wide open, but there is a delay in the sound?)

So guess who had to do the consoling? Me! (Ain't something wrong with this picture?)

I hugged Kevin and quietly kept repeating, "I am not going anywhere. God is not through with me yet."

After Kevin got it together, he and I hurriedly left the office. We had to pick up the boys from school. Because we wanted to go together, he followed me home so that I could drop off my car.

While on my way to the house, it soon dawned on me that my husband was *not* supposed to be there when I first received the news. Both of Kevin's parents had died from a form of cancer. His mother had died of Hodgkin's disease when he was 9, and his dad had died of lung cancer just right after we had married. I concluded that part of my new assignment was to reflect another outcome of cancer for Kevin—survival. Lord knows, I didn't welcome this new responsibility, but I knew that God wouldn't give me an assignment that I could not complete.

When I finally got into Kevin's car, we rode in silence. We were both deep in thought. Finally he asked, "Cynthia, who do you want to tell? You know we don't have to share this with anyone, if you don't want."

"Well, I know that I don't want to tell the boys right now," I answered immediately. "Our sensitive Julien would not be able to handle it, and Justen is too young to understand."

After contemplating his question a few more minutes, I then said, "I do think that I want to share this with my family and friends. Kevin, if I ever needed prayer, I need it now, and folks can't pray for me if they don't know."

He agreed, and so ended any further discussion of this matter for the rest of the evening. Our eldest, Julien, was approaching the car. Thus, for the remainder of the evening we tried our best to conduct ourselves with some degree of normalcy around the boys. Indeed, I believe we were both contenders for an Academy Award that night!

October 17, 2006

I left for work the next morning in a state of bewilderment. After a very restless night, I awoke to the stark reality of my new situation. What in the world was I about to face?

Surgery, radiation, chemotherapy? Ah, come on. This is unreal!

"Good morning, Cynthia, how are you today?" Susan asked in her familiarly pleasant manner when I passed by her desk.

"I am good. How are you?" I answered and continued to my office. I closed the door behind me, placed my coat and bag in their customary places, and sat at my desk. Paralyzed.

After about ten minutes of being in a motionless state, I abruptly returned back to Susan's desk and sat down.

"You got a minute?" I asked.

"Sure, what's up?" she asked.

I began coolly, "Well, I thought that I would give you a little heads up on what to expect for the rest of the semester. Some things have changed." I paused and a little more unsteadily said, "And I remember you saying a few weeks back that you were a Christian, and so I thought that maybe you could keep me in your prayers as well." At this point, as you can imagine, I was emotionally starting to come loose at the seams.

"Cynthia, what's wrong?" Susan asked as she came from around her desk to sit down beside me.

Now, for the third time in twenty-four hours, I again spoke the words, "I have breast cancer."

They say that the third time is the charm, right? Well, I am no exception. I was done! You could have stuck a pin in me and I would have popped. And now, the very same woman who months before I didn't even know if we would get along, was holding my hand and asking to pray with me right then and there.

"Please," I replied and we went to my office.

Can I say that the sister prayed? Or, can I more appropriately say that the sister implored the throne of the kingdom on my behalf?!

Behind the closed doors of my office that morning, Susan prayed and I released. It was as if I had specifically outlined to her every fear, doubt and worry that had crept into my spirit since getting the news. And as she articulated every one of them to God and asked for His removal of them, I literally felt as if a burden was being lifted after each appeal. It was one of the most emotionally and spiritually cleansing moments that I had had in years.

Afterwards, we laughed and cried together. We laughed about how uncomfortable we initially were about our new assignments in this move. Susan joked about how she struggled with the idea of additional responsibilities, and I quipped about how resistive I was to being in the office with another headstrong woman. Then, Susan offered one of the most profound insights of my journey to date.

"Cynthia, we thought that we had finally had this all figured out. The idea was to have me manage your calendar to assist in your academic advising, right? Well, little did we know that way back in April, God was setting things up so that I would be able to manage your calendar for another reason. He knew that by my managing your calendar, I would then know when your doctor's appointments were. And if I knew when your doctors' appointments were, I would also know when specifically to pray for you."

Talk about God's providence. A simple office move, huh? Who would have thought.

Pass the tissues, please.

….Oh, and let me throw in a footnote here. You know, both Kevin and I went to work that day, or so I thought. I got a phone call in my office later that morning from my mother.

"Cindy, you need to check in on Kevin. He is not doing well."

"Well, what do you mean?" I asked. "Have you talked to him or something?"

"Yes, Kevin called me quite upset."

"He called you from work?"

"No, he is at home."

"At home? We both left the house this morning for work."

"Girl, just check up on your husband," my mom replied and hung up.

"Lord, what is going on with Kevin? He seemed to be doing fine when he left this morning," I thought while dialing his cell phone.

"Hello," he answered.

"Kevin, where are you?"

"At home," he snickered.

"What are you doing at home?"

He began, "Well, Cynthia, I'm not like you. I need time to process."

"Okay…"

"I was at school and just got overwhelmed. For a little while I was hiding behind my computer at my desk trying to give instruction to the students so they couldn't see the tears streaming down my face." He paused and then laughed.

"Cynthia, imagine me trying to give direction to the orchestra kids from behind my desk— '1-2-ready-go'—that was just not working. I couldn't let them see me like this, so I took the remainder of the day off."

"And you called mom?" I asked teasingly.

"Yep, I talked to your mom, your dad, Aunt Edith, and anybody else I could reach. I was some kind of bad off. In fact, Cynthia, I was so bad off that when I got home, I let out a holla in the house that scared me. I didn't even know that I could make a sound like that!"

We were both laughing quite hard at this point.

He continued, "I even called my boy, Tony. I was crying so hard that I had to stop and tell him that even though I was crying, I was no punk. I just loved my wife. I just loved my wife, man."

My stomach was hurting. Thank God for laughter! Even in the midst of this difficult time, God was still allowing Kevin and me to find the humor in things. Boy, I can't stress enough how much laughter is important in keeping your spiritual sanity and emotional health.

Then a more serious Kevin shared, "God did reveal to me one thing as I was processing."

"Really, what?"

"That you are going to be alright," He said. "You know, up until now, I have known Him only as a Comforter when it has come to cancer and my family. However, this go-around, I believe that He is going to show Himself to me as a Healer."

Okay, do you recall my thoughts when returning home from the doctor's office? Will someone now please pass the tissue *box*!

3
CHAPTER

"And God said, Let there be light: and there was light. And God saw the light, that it was good: and God divided the light from the darkness. And God called the light Day, and the darkness he called Night. And the evening and the morning were the first day."
Genesis 1: 3-5

When the light of truth illuminates our dark conditions, will we be able to stand the view?

From: Cynthia
Sent: Thu 11/16/2006 12:42 AM
To: Prayer Sisters
Subject: RE(2): For we wrestle not against flesh and blood...
(ROUND 1)

My Praying Sisters,

I have never known a more concerned group of women than you!
I am not complaining, though. It is great to feel so much love
(*smile*). Truly, I am doing well. I am feeding on the Word
spiritually and on organic whole foods physically. The Word-
not a problem, but really, no one could have ever told me that I
could, first of all, endure sipping on raw broccoli, carrot, and
spinach juices (I would barely eat them cooked a month ago). But
that is exactly what I am doing, and actually enjoying it. So that
means you all have really been holding me up in prayer because
this diet change in itself is a miracle!

Yes, my sisters, I am drinking wheatgrass juice in the morning
followed by breakfast that often includes Ezekiel bread and a
cottage cheese/flax oil/fruit juice mixture. Throughout the day,
you may find me sipping on broccoli and pineapple juice or
carrot and apple juice. Foods of choice these days are sweet
potatoes, lentils, beans, tuna, salmon, and leafy veggies of all
types. My snacks of choice these days are raw sunflower
seeds/raisin mix, stone whole wheat crackers with hummus, and
fruit. I even find a way to get in one clove of garlic daily. Ha!
For those of you who knew my diet before, you are likely shaking
your heads in disbelief. Yes, I have not tasted refined sugar,
enriched flour, or hydrogenated fats for three weeks.

Consequently, I have lost 10 lbs., my complexion is the best it
has ever been, and I feel fit for the battle. My poor boys are
wondering, though, what is going on. Julien, my 8 yr. old son,
now often asks," have we become health food nuts or something?" Just today he asked me why do we keep buying organ

stuff (he meant "organic") LOL! Poor Kevin (my hubby), he has joined me in my "change in diet" campaign and has lost nearly 15 lbs. that he was not trying to lose (because he was small-framed from the beginning). So he is feeling a bit self-conscious (keep a brother in prayer *smile*). My youngest, 4-yr.old Justen—well, we argue every morning because he does not like the "new" juice (fresh orange/carrot/pineapple juice) because it does not look "good." Mind you, he has yet to taste it. Y'all, now, this juice is good, for real! Instead, he insists on wanting the "old" juice (that has 23 grams of refined sugar in it) because as he puts it, "it makes him feel better." (Whatever that means.)

Thus, I just want you to know that while I am not too excited about surgery on this coming Monday (Nov. 20), I am prayed up and feel physically prepared. Your prayers, cards, well-wishes, and phone calls have truly sustained me during this waiting period. I have had my moments, but EVERY time I have had one of them, God has placed me on one of your hearts and I have received an email, a card, flowers, or a phone call from one of you. And you know what? That's just like God to always remind me that He is here with me via His angels on earth (you). Hence, while I may have not individually responded to all of your messages, do know that I have gotten each and every one, and I thank you.

For those of you who have inquired about any needed help during my surgery and recovery, along with Kevin, my mother and sister will be in town during my surgery. Further, my whole family~ parents, siblings, and in-laws will be in town with me for Thanksgiving, but feel free to call to see if there is any additional help needed.

Also, I have unearthed some gems of knowledge regarding overall diet and health that I would love to share with you more fully later.

Lastly, some of you have asked about the exact time of my surgery on Monday. I won't know for certain until this Friday. I will let you know then. I do know though, that I will be at the hospital until Tuesday. I will not know any results from the surgery, however, until a week after the surgery. To be specific, I meet with my oncologist to discuss the results (i.e., what stage is the cancer, what treatments I should consider, etc.) on Tuesday, Nov. 28.

Well, that should do it for now. My prayer requests have not changed, so please continue to keep these requests lifted. Thank you.

Love your sis,
Cynthia

Okay, I have to own up to something. The lump under my arm was not the only abnormal thing that the doctor found during my annual physical. Not only did several other routine tests come back atypical, I also found out that I was walking around with pneumonia. You heard me, pneumonia!

Thus, as I pondered over just how I got to this physical low in my life, I swiftly realized that I needed to reconsider my current working definition of spiritual darkness. This would prove to be critical in my ability to make application of God's Creation to my present trek.

Prior to this episode in my life, when I tended to think of spiritual darkness, I generally focused on the sins of the flesh as described in Galatians 5:19-21—lust, greed, jealousy, hatred, deceit, adultery, fornication, addiction, etc. Thus, I must admit that my study of the Creation was a bit perplexing from Day One. In particular, I was stumped as to how God's dividing light from darkness had anything to do with what I was going through. I did consider the notion of whether God led me to this passage to reflect on some sin of the past. However, I quickly moved away from this train of thought when I could not see how my having breast cancer could cast light on any of my past transgressions (or at least, those that I could remember—you know we have ways of forgetting things that we don't want to remember). I even entertained the idea that Day One was metaphorical for the beginning of a new day in my life. And while I could see some application in certain areas of my current journey, I was sincerely hoping that this was not the case, for this was not how I wanted to start a new chapter in my life.

I then decided to look up the formal definition of darkness. Interestingly, of the definitions that I read, the one that grabbed my attention was, "opaque in nature; dim; dull in color." As I further mulled over this definition, God began to bring to mind other traits that reflect forms of darkness—denial, avoidance, ignorance, ambition (we call it blind sometimes, don't we?) and idealism, just to name a few. All of these attributes can dull our view of reality, and lead to significant collateral damage in our lives, if not careful. In my case, I think it was a combination of more than a few, and so here is where the light piercing began for me.

What

Take a "do whatever is needed" spirit and a "make it happen" attitude, and generally what do you get? Things done? Yes. Goals accomplished? Yes. Now, add good intentions (about a cup). Then add noble goals (one quart). Sounds good, doesn't it? Now, add denial of rest (about a half-gallon). Then stir in ignorance of the affects of stress (about two liters), and generously sprinkle in the avoidance of "because-they-don't-taste-as-good-and-cost-too-much" healthy foods. Set timer for about twenty years and simmer. After ten years of simmering, add one husband. Around about the 12 year-interval and 16 year-interval, add a son. Finally, throw in a couple of handfuls of failures, disappointments, and heartaches. Then, add to taste, exercise-when-convenient habits, and there you have it—*The Cynthia Turner Soup* (pre-October 16, 2006).

Funny, right? But can anyone else relate to these traits and tendencies? Perhaps not. Maybe, instead, you possess a codependent trait (i.e., unable to assert yourself healthily in relationships for fear of angering/hurting/losing the other). Consequently, you consistently find yourself in dysfunctional relationships that involve a lot of ignorant behavior and subsequent stressing, denying and avoiding to keep such behavior to a minimum.

Or perhaps, you may have a propensity to look at life from a lens of ideals—the ideal job, the ideal spouse, the ideal children, the ideal weight, the ideal beauty, the ideal home, and so on and so on. As a result, you find yourself doing a lot of stressing, denying, and avoiding trying to aim at moving targets.

Whatever the case may be, I have concluded that, over time, these traits, when not kept in check, rack up significant damages that are deeply penetrating and far-reaching. Further, when light pierces these opaque areas in our lives (which it always does sooner or later), we are all too often caught off-guard and shocked of the magnitude of the costs. In some cases, broken relationships. In some cases, troubled children. In my case, ailing health.

Now, let's revisit my initial question. How can one walk around with his/her body literally breaking down and not know it? Easily. As for me, I just had too much on my plate. Sleep had become a luxury rather than a need during this time (denial). Eating? Well, I ate when I could, and as healthily as I knew how to (you will find out in chapter ten that I was greatly in the dark in this area—ignorance). I made sure (or so I thought) that my husband and children got what they needed. But as for tending to myself, in my mind it was all about making the sacrifices now for the great payoff later (idealism). At the time, I was so focused on achieving seemingly honorable goals (ambition) that I was totally oblivious to any changes in my physical well-being.

So actually October 16, 2006 was a dawning of a new day for me. And once God cast light on these opaque traits of mine, He made it quite difficult for me slip back into my nighttime tendencies. How? Check out some of the stories that coincidentally (ha!) made news during the span of my journey:

Younger African American Women At Significantly Higher Risk For Breast Cancer
(11 Nov 2006) Source: Breast Cancer News
Although white women have the highest overall breast cancer incidence rates, African-American women under age 40 have a significantly higher incidence of breast cancer as well as a higher rate of death from breast cancer than do white women. Furthermore, African-Americans with breast cancer die at a younger age than women in other groups.

Health Behaviors and Breast Cancer: Experiences of Urban African American Women
(2006) Source: Health Education & Behavior, Vol. 33, No. 5
Breast-cancer survival rates are lower among African-American women compared to White women. Obesity may contribute to this disparity. African-American women have the highest rates of being overweight or obese compared to all other groups in the U.S. Specifically, 77% (three out of every four African-American women) are overweight or obese (compared to 61% nationally). Obesity increases risk of recurrence.

Food Choice and Obesity in Black America: Creating a New Cultural Diet
(2006) Author: Eric J. Bailey (Praeger Publishers)
Book examines, among other things, the traditional African-American diet known as "soul food" which tends to be low in fiber, high in fat, sodium, nitrates, sugar, and/or cholesterol, and

discuss its negative impact on health-related issues prevalent in the African-American community such as obesity, diabetes, cancer and heart disease.

Frequent Fast Food Meals Pack on Pounds
(22 Oct 2007) Source: medpagetoday.com
According to study, dining on fast food three or more times a week translated into as much as four extra pounds compared with less frequent consumption. Latino-Americans and African-Americans frequented fast food places most often, dining out 6.7 and 6.2 times a week, respectively.
(Similar to traditional "soul food," fast food tends to be low in fiber, high in fat, sodium, nitrates, sugar, and/or cholesterol.)

Diet and Cancer Prevention
(2006) Source: British Nutrition Foundation
Researchers posit that approximately 30% of cancers can be prevented by dietary means in the Western countries. They further submit that being physically active can reduce the risk of certain cancers by 30-50%.

The big 3: foods that may fight cancer: pile your plate high with fruits, vegetables, and whole grains and it may help you avoid breast, ovarian, and colon cancer
(Nov 2006) Source: Food & Fitness Advisor
Scientific evidence is mounting that a diet composed mostly of fruits, vegetables and grains—coupled with regular exercise and weight control—can help lower your risk of cancer, and can also cut the risk of a cancer recurrence.

Workouts Help Ward Off Cancer's Return
(30 Nov 2006) Source: Healthday News
In an update of nutrition and physical activity recommendations for cancer survivors, the American Cancer Society conclude that exercising and maintaining a healthy weight are important factors in preventing malignancy's return, at least for some forms of the disease.

Diet And Exercise Key To Surviving Breast Cancer

(11 June 2007) Source: Science Daily

Results from a new longitudinal study from the Moores Cancer Center at the University of California, San Diego (UCSD) suggest that breast cancer survivors who eat a healthy diet and exercise moderately can reduce their risk of dying from breast cancer by half, regardless of their weight.

Depression, stress, and blood pressure in urban African-American women

(Spring 2006) Source: Journal of Progress in Cardiovascular Nursing

Results suggest that African-American women have disturbingly high rates of hypertension, exceeding all other ethnic groups, including African-American men.

Stress and Gender

(2006) Source: Consumer Health Interactive

In a 2006 survey conducted by the American Psychological Association (APA), researchers found that women felt more stressed out than men did. Specifically, 51% of women reported that stress had an impact on their lives, compared to 43% of men. African-American women were the highest group concerned about stress.

Stress and cancer

(3 Nov 2006) Source: Science Daily

A new report reveals how norepinephrine, a hormone produced during bouts of stress, accelerates the formation of more tumors and stimulate the release of a compound in tumor cells, facilitating the growth of new blood cells that feed cancer cells.

Stress: A Cause of Cancer?

(10 Dec 2006) Source: psychcentral.com

Increasing evidence indicate some link between stress and developing certain kinds of cancer, as well as how the disease progresses.

You Sleep Less Than You Think
(6 July 2006) Source: cbsnews.com

In a long-term study of heart disease, researchers strapped sensitive movement detectors to the wrists of volunteers ranging in age from 38- to 50-years old. They measured how long people slept, how long it took them to get to sleep, how much time they spent in bed, and how much of their time in bed they slept. Among other things, results revealed that African-Americans' sleep duration (men: 5.1 hours; women- 5.9 hours) was significantly shorter than that of Caucasians (men- 6.1 hours; women- 6.9 hours). These differences persisted even when taking into consideration socioeconomic, employment, household, and lifestyle factors. Lower income, however, was associated with taking longer to get to sleep and lower sleep efficiency.

All wound up over lack of sleep
(4 Nov 2006) Source: The Daily Telegraph

Researchers suggest that there are links between inadequate sleep (less than six hours of sleep a night) and health illnesses such as colds and flu, hypertension, diabetes, obesity and cancer. Mounting evidence indicate that poor sleep weakens the body's immune system, which in turn affects hormone production and increases the chance of one becoming ill and developing chronic health problems. In one study, the American Cancer Society followed the sleep habits of more than a million people over a six-year period. Among other things, it found that those who slept about 7 hours a night had the best chances of surviving cancer. The worst survival rate was among those who slept less than 4.5 hours. (Interestingly, similar mortality rates were found for those who got too much sleep—nine hours or more.)

Sleep: It's required
(24 Oct 2006) Source: Los Angeles Times

Studies show that adequate sleep (7 to 8 hours a night) is as crucial to a healthy life as diet and exercise, particularly when it comes to obesity, diabetes, and other chronic illnesses. However, according to a 2005 survey by the National Sleep Foundation, about 40 percent of people in the U.S. say they average fewer than seven hours of sleep, and about 71 percent indicate that they average fewer than eight hours of sleep. In one longitudinal study, researchers found that after 12 to 16 years, women who slept, on average, less than five hours per night were 5 1/2 pounds heavier than those who slept an average of seven hours nightly.

Now how's that for some Heavenly illumination!

CHAPTER 4

"And God said, Let there be a firmament in the midst of the waters, and let it divide the waters from the waters. And God made the firmament, and divided the waters which were under the firmament from the waters which were above the firmament: and it was so. And God called the firmament Heaven. And the evening and the morning were the second day." Genesis 1: 6-8

To not consider our life's battles from an aerial position is to give our foe the chance to defeat us from **every** position.

From: Cynthia
Sent: Wed 11/22/2006 11:35 AM
To: Prayer Sisters
Subject: ROUND 2: For we wrestle not against flesh and blood...

Victory is mine...victory is mine...My praying sisters, God is FAITHFUL! I am home resting (and have been since 1pm on yesterday, Tuesday). You know I wanted to email you then, but in obedience to my family~ particularly HUSBAND and MOTHER, I waited until today.

Well, what can I say? There are so many, but I will share all of it with you later. However, what I will say is that the doctors removed the tumor and surrounding tissue as well as several lymph nodes. More importantly, here is what the doctors had to say:

1) Victory shout #1: The tumor was smaller than initially measured—the surgeon indicated that when he went to remove the tumor it was surrounded and covered by a clot of blood. He suggested that a likely explanation was that this clot of blood was scar tissue that resulted from the biopsy. The problem with this explanation is that they measured my tumor BEFORE the biopsy. My explanation: "The prayers of the righteous availeth much." (In fact, my mom said it best when she said that the doctor did not realize that he was talking spiritually when he said that my tumor was covered by BLOOD~ he just did not know whose BLOOD he was referring to!)

2) Victory shout #2: The doctors thought that they would have to cut me in two places: one to remove the tumor and another to remove the lymph nodes...Only one cut was made, and the surgeon was able to do both. Moreover, he removed fewer lymph nodes than expected.

3) Victory shout #3: The doctors had forewarned me of likely side effects of the surgery such as nausea; pain, tingling and

numbness in the arm and hand where the lymph nodes were removed; and possible lymphedema (swelling and limited activity of the arm). Now, while lymphedema will always be concern for me for the rest of my life (y'all pray with me against this), I ate like a queen yesterday, and I am typing this email message like it was the day before surgery.

I will know the results of the testing of the tissue (which determines the stage of the cancer and treatment plan) on Tuesday, Nov. 28th. So again, I ask that you all continue to pray the following:

1) *The lymph node results will come back negative of any cancer (this determines whether the cancer has likely spread).*
2) *The doctors will accurately assess my pathology report from the surgery and we will determine the treatment that will CURE my cancer.*
3) *I will continue to experience no ill side effects or complications from surgery.*
4) *Lymphedema will never be a condition that I experience.*
5) *My family and I will continue to remain at peace throughout this process.*
6) *My boys will continue to not be ill-affected by this process.*
7) *I will continue to receive the best doctor care on this side of Jordan.*

God is good, y'all. I will keep you posted. I love y'all so. Your prayers have been, well...WOW! Now, though, I will get back to bed before my mother gets on my case. Have a blessed Thanksgiving! Know that I will.

Love,
Cynthia

From: Cynthia
Sent: Fri 11/24/2006 2:08 PM
To: Prayer Sisters
Subject: RE(2): ROUND 2: For we wrestle not against flesh and blood...

Sisters,

If you're going to be a soldier, sometimes you've got to be on the front line and experience the battle ...

Just had preliminary discussion with the surgeon regarding the pathology report (i.e., surgery results). I will have to undergo further surgery (re-excision). While the tumor was small, it was deeper than initially thought. Hence, they have to go back in and cut out the remainder of the tumor which has found its way in the underlying muscle tissue. This will take place in the next week or two. Results from testing of the lymph nodes found cancer in only 1 of 11 nodes (the one closest to the tumor), which is good, but now means that I will likely need to consider chemotherapy along with radiation. However, the key part of our conversation this morning was that my cancer was COMPLETELY CURABLE.

Again, I will know further when I talk with the oncologist (the cancer specialist) on Tuesday. But know that I know that our God is ABLE and WILLING to heal me, and I am TOTALLY confident that He will take me through this process, making me a better and stronger person physically, emotionally, and spiritually in the end.

Keep sending up the prayers, and I will keep you posted. While the timeline has changed, victory still is MINE!(Y'all know that, right?) Love y'all!

-Cynthia

From: Cynthia
Sent: Fri 12/1/2006 10:13 AM
To: Prayer Sisters
Subject: ROUND 3: For we wrestle not against flesh and blood...

My Praying Sisters,

As you are aware, I met with my oncologist and surgeon (again) this past Tuesday to further assess my surgery results (pathology report). As earlier reported, I will have to undergo further surgery (re-excision). The next surgery date is Monday, Dec. 18. It is expected to be outpatient surgery. (I will return home Monday evening.) Because they expect to cut into some muscle tissue this go around to make certain they have removed the entire tumor, they are suggesting that my recovery may be a little more uncomfortable (i.e., painful) and longer this go around, but you know that I am not claiming that! Further, after my full recovery from surgery, my oncologist and I have discussed a possible plan beginning sometime in January of 4 mos. of chemotherapy followed by 6 weeks of radiation. However, there are several tests that we are still awaiting results to conclusively determine the treatment plan. She again reiterated that my cancer was COMPLETELY CURABLE.

Until the remaining test results come back next week, I am going to wait to give you my next specific prayer requests. However, know that I am doing well. Of course, as you may ~~would~~ expect, I did struggle for a moment with the expected treatment plan. I really wanted this event to be a 50-yd. dash because I've always held up pretty good in short distance events (*smile*). However, God reminded me that "the race is not given to the swift or the strong, but to the one that endureth until the end." Thus, while I know that I am assured the victory in this battle, I am just now realizing that, among other things, God is just simply building me up to be a marathon runner for Him because He needs more marathon running saints on the battlefield (and we won't volunteer! LOL).

Until the next update...

Love ya,
Cynthia

From: Turner, Cynthia
Sent: Fri 12/1/2006 10:26 AM
TO: Prayer Sisters
Subject: RE: ROUND 3: For we wrestle not against flesh and blood....

By the way, y'all, I plan to have a big PRAISE party BEFORE and AFTER my chemo and radiation treatment process next year. Any folks willing to be on the planning committee? Holla...

Love,
Cynthia

𝓗ave you ever gone into a fight confident of a quick knock-out, but soon realize that instead you will have to go all twelve rounds? As you can see in the preceding series of email messages, that very scenario played out for me in real time when I was told of the results of my lumpectomy. Here is a little more of how I discovered the full strength of my foe.

The Call

The phone rang late Friday morning, the day after Thanksgiving. I expected the call to be a holiday greeting from a family member or friend and was quite surprised to recognize it to be from my surgeon's office. My surgeon told me that he likely would not know the results of the tests from surgery until the following Monday. So, what was he doing calling me today?

"Hello, may I speak to Cynthia Turner?" a male voice requested as I picked up the phone.

"This is she."

"Hello, Cynthia, this is Dr. Smith.[1] Did I catch you at a bad time?" he asked.

"No, this is fine," I tried to answer calmly.

"Well, I have the pathology report from your recent surgery, and wanted to share with you the results."

"Okay," I quietly respond. (Oh, Lord, here it comes.)

"Actually, the results are a mixed bag of sorts," he replied.

"Really?" (Dear Lord, can I handle this?)

"Yes," he continued (as well as I can remember), "it seems that while the tumor was smaller than initially measured, it was deeper than we thought. Consequently, I am not comfortable with the margins we cleared around the deepest edge of the tumor. So I would like to go in and perform additional surgery to ensure that we get a clear margin in that area. Further, the results of the testing of cancer in the lymph nodes reveal 1 of the 11 lymph nodes removed to be positive. Oddly enough, however, the lymph node that tested positive was not the sentinel node (the first lymph node that cancer cells will generally spread to after breaking away from the main cancer in the breast). In fact, the cancer jumped over the sentinel and the three closest axillary nodes to the tumor and showed up in the fourth axillary node."

"What does this mean? Is this unusual?" I was almost holding my breath.

"Well, a better word is 'uncommon.' We see this in only 5% of the cases, but that just tells you how unpredictable of an animal that cancer is," he responded.

Silence. I don't know what to think now.

After a slight pause, he followed, "I see that you meet with your oncologist on Tuesday, right?"

"Yes, but question—does this mean that I will have to undergo chemotherapy?" I asked.

"Well, at this point, your oncologist will be able to discuss with you the alternative treatment plans. Chemotherapy and radiation are generally the standard treatment when cancer is found in the lymph nodes, even in the case of only one, but she will be better able to discuss this with you and help you weigh your options," he answered.

Feeling my anxiety, he then said, "Cynthia, while this may not be completely what you wanted to hear, the good news is that your situation is one where the prognosis is excellent for total cure with the appropriate treatment. Might you have any questions of me?"

"No, not at the moment."

He then told me to telephone his nurse next week to schedule my next surgery date, we exchanged goodbyes, and so ended the call.

Boy, talk about scrambling to my corner to regroup! Another surgery? Radiation?! Chemotherapy?!! Honestly, at that point, I wanted to turn in my "grown-up" card, and go back to being the little Cindy whose biggest health struggle was swallowing allergy pills. (Ha! I know that when I was growing up my mom must have wanted to hurt me sometimes. I had severe allergies and often had to take allergy medicine. For some reason, I couldn't figure out how to get that pill in just the right place in my mouth to get it to go down when I swallowed. As a consequence, many times I gagged. Other times, I choked. I even threw up on an occasion or two. In my defense, though, don't forget that, back in my day, medicine for children was not as tasty as it is nowadays! Now that I think about it, was children medicine even made back then? Or, did we just take half the dosage of the grownup medicine? If my memory serves me correctly, I do recall my mom cutting my pills in half...)

In any case, as I grappled with this latest news, I wasn't certain how to respond. I was still confident of victory, but gosh, did I have to go through all of that? Just a few weeks before, my biggest concern was about extending my days in high heels. Now overnight, I was being told that I must focus on extending my days, period! My spiritual calm had now been replaced with fevered apprehension. My mind was reeling. Another surgery meant more time off from my responsibilities. Who would take over my classes, and how well would my household manage during this time? Further, let's not begin to entertain the idea of chemo and radiation. That meant being sick, losing hair, more time off from work, and more concerns about the children and hubby. I just wasn't ready to process all of these new developments.

And so, I didn't. That's right. I told my family what the doctor said, and then emotionally clocked out. I called a "timeout."

By the way, did I tell you that I have a beautiful family? Well, I do. When my parents and three siblings learned of my surgery date and realized that it was close to the Thanksgiving holiday, all of them (including spouses) decided to fly to Champaign to be with me and my family for Thanksgiving. A family first. Wasn't that wonderful?

Getting back. Of course, when I shared with my family the latest, they were concerned about how I was feeling. Truthfully, I am not sure how I responded. Was I overwhelmed? Yes. Numb? Probably. Was I ready to engage in thoughtful discussion about it? Nope. You see, I quickly realized that my head was not in the right place. I had allowed the news to rattle me so much so that I had peeked at my battle through my weak and feeble human spectacles, and the visual was frightening!

I recall the house being quiet for some time after I shared the doctor's report. I believe that everyone sensed my need for a "timeout" and tried to respect it as I attempted to gather my thoughts. And as He always does when I begin to unravel, God began to speak into my spirit.

"The twelve spies," He whispered. Immediately I went to my Bible and revisited the story of the twelve spies who Moses had sent to survey the promised land of Canaan for the Israelites (see Numbers 14). God told the Israelites that Canaan was rich and fertile. And upon returning, all of the spies did indeed confirm this when giving their account. They even brought back a piece of fruit from the land to provide evidence. Nonetheless, when ten of the spies presented their outlook on the prospects of entering the land (*that God had promised*), they shifted their focus to the size of their giant opponents, losing sight of the breadth of their God's omnipotence. (Seeing any parallels? Lord, I was!)

But God reminded me, that this was the report of the ten. What did the other two say? (I am about to get happy, folks!) Well Caleb, one of the two, said, "We should go up and take possession of the land, for we can certainly do it." (Numbers 14:30, NIV)

It was if God was asking me at that point, what position was I going to take in my battle—the position of the majority whose focus was on the circumstances on the ground? Or, the position of the minority whose focus was on the power source above? In response, I wrote the preceding email message to my prayer sisters that Friday afternoon which began, "If you're going to be a soldier, sometimes you've got to be on the front line and experience the battle..."

CHAPTER 5

"And God said, Let the waters under heaven be gathered together unto one place, and let the dry land appear: and it was so. And God called the dry land Earth; and the gathering together of the waters called He Seas: and God saw that it was good. And God said, Let the earth bring forth grass, the herb yielding seed, and the fruit tree yielding fruit after his kind, whose seed is in itself, upon the earth: and it was so. And the earth brought forth grass, and herb yielding seed after his kind, and the tree yielding fruit, whose seed was in itself, after his kind: and God saw that it was good. And the evening and the morning were the third day." Genesis 1: 9-13

Because God's people are a peculiar people, the fruit they yield ought naturally be distinct.

From: Cynthia
Sent: Fri 12/15/2006 2:35 PM
To: Prayer Sisters
Subject: ROUND 4: For we wrestle not against flesh and blood...

Okay, sisters, here we go again. The next surgery date is this
Monday, Dec. 18. TIME: 7:30AM. It is expected to be outpatient surgery. (I will return home Monday evening.) No more
lymph nodes will be removed (not needed, praise the Lord!). It is
now just a matter of the doctor going in again and getting a clean
margin around one edge of the former tumor. FYI: When
removing tumors, in general, surgeons like to be certain that they
have completely removed a tumor by cutting an area around the
tumor that is void of tumor cells (what is known as clean
margins). Generally, however, they don't know with certainty if
they have accomplished this until after reviewing the post-op
surgery results. In my case, my first surgery results indicated that
there was one side of the breast tissue removed where the tumor
reached the tissue's edges. Thus, they are going back in to
remove a bit more of breast tissue (and some surrounding muscle
tissue) in that area to get a clean margin there. Got it? Okay,
here are my prayer requests this go around:

1) During my hospital stay, God will cover and protect me.
*2) God will guide the hands of the operating doctor, and the doctor will
successfully get clean margins (allowing this to be my last surgery needed).*
*3) I will experience no ill side effects or any complications from this
surgery.*
4) I will recover as quickly from this surgery as I did from the first.
*5) The doctors will accurately assess my pathology report (surgery results)
and determine the treatment that will remove any and all remaining
cancer cells that may have gotten into my bloodstream. That is, the
medical treatment determined will completely cure me of cancer.*
*6) Those who surround me will only speak life and victory over this event
to and for me. (Can I stick a pin here for a second? *smile*~ You will be
amazed of some of the things that have come out of folks' mouths thinking
that they are encouraging me! My biggest battle, thus far, has truly been*

trying to ward off the doom-and-gloom spirits some folks have uncon-
sciously been putting on me. Yes, my circumstance is unfortunate, and,
yes, it doesn't make sense for someone my age. I have learned from past
trials, though, that when things just don't make sense, once I accept the
circumstance but release its' outcome to God, my complete surrender
creates the perfect stage for God to show up and show out! And since I
have experienced Him show out before, why would I doubt that He
would do so again?! So pleez pray this point fervently for me. Thank
you.) Okay, now continuing (*smile*)...
7) God will continue to give me and my family peace during this event.
8) My boys will continue to not be in any way ill-affected by this process.
9) I will represent God well.

That should do it for now. I will update you on the other side of
surgery.

Love,
Cynthia

P.S. My mom will be back (YEAH!), so I should be okay again
this time around, but feel free to check in. Also, make certain
that you have marked Saturday, Jan. 6 in your calendars (date of
my before (chemo) praise party). More info to follow.

From: Cynthia
Sent: Wed 12/20/2006 7:27 AM
TO: Prayer Sisters
Subject: RE: ROUND 4: For we wrestle not against flesh and
blood...

God is good, y'all, you know that right? I have been home since
Monday. In fact, the hospital released me so fast, I didn't even
get a meal before I left, just some crackers (LOL). (I was home
even before my boys returned home from school.) I would have
emailed earlier (you know me), but they gave me some antibiotics
(to prevent any possible infection) and pain medicine that have
been keeping me extra sleepy. So I have been resting. I have had
minimal to no pain~ of course, that is the result of nothing but

God, and your prayers! Again, I thank you SO much for your prayers!

I don't know much else until the results come back within the next day or two. I will update you further then.

Love ya,
Cynthia

From: Cynthia
Sent: Fri 12/22/2006 4:12 PM
To: Prayer Sisters
Subject: My Christmas Gift

HAL-LE-LU-JAH!! Surgery results show no residual tumor and margins are now clear. Besides the birth of Jesus Christ, this is, by far, the next-best Christmas gift I have ever received. (I should know of my chemo treatment plan by the end of the next week and will update you then.) Y'all have a good Christmas. My family and I plan to!

Love,
Cynthia

One thing I do know for certain. Serious illness (or loss) will cause us to acknowledge the brevity [shortness] of life. Furthermore, it will often cause us to assess our productivity (fruitfulness) to date. I, being no different, began to take a hard look at my life accomplishments roughly about this stage of the battle. And curiously, it began with the following short story that God placed on my heart late one evening when studying His third day of creation. As I notated this story, it prompted me to consider my "life performance" against the backdrop of this powerful day. It is as follows.

> There was once a 4-year old little girl who had just discovered that she was soon to have a baby brother. A bit concerned about this news, she subsequently asked her mother whether mommies could have baby animals. The puzzled mother sat the young girl down and shared with her that no, mommies could not birth baby animals for this was unnatural. The mother went on to explain that like an apple can only carry apple seeds, mommies could only carry human seeds. Later that night as the young pre-schooler prayed, she said, "Dear God, I know what mommy said, but I know if You can let a man live in a whale's belly, You can let an animal live in a human mommy's belly. So could You please put a baby pony in my mommy's stomach because I really want a pony and not a brother."

Cute, right? However, the power of this story for me was in its revelation concerning God's third day of creation. Follow, if you will. Again, Genesis 1:11-13 says that on the third day, "…God said, Let the earth bring forth grass, the herb yielding seed, and the *fruit tree yielding fruit after his kind*, whose seed is in itself, upon the earth: and it was so. And the earth brought forth grass, and *herb yielding seed after his kind*, and the *tree yielding fruit, whose seed was in itself, after his kind*: and God saw that it was good."

As I studied these verses in the context of the "pony" tale, I soon discerned a principle that I had not recognized before. That is, by God's design, He purposed His creation to yield fruit only of its kind. As the scriptures indicate, He saw this to be good. Consequently, I surmised that God must have then intended for us to labor in areas that employ our individual gifts, talents and experiences. By operating in these fertile environments, we correspondingly put in to motion our ability and capability to impart to this life our own unique contributions (i.e., produce fruit of our own kind).

Have you ever considered the breathtaking splendor of God's landscape we know as nature? The brilliance of its colors. The plethora of its textures and shapes. The purity of its fragrances and aromas. This artistry is no result of some homogeneous production mill. This masterpiece is the outcome of each individual plant and tree, big and small, contributing its own distinct garden. Such a revelation brought to bear the following question for me as I reflected upon my life achievements to date: have I been properly "tending my garden"?

To answer this, I first had to toss out all of my learned notions of achievement and accomplishment. Specifically, I had to rethink the value I attached to conformity and assimilation. But wow, that proved to be tough for me. We live in a world that applauds people's ability to mimic others' deeds and represent worldly ideals. We exist in a society that rewards persons' abilities to reproduce others' successes and replicate others' feats.

But at this point of deliberation, God moved me to simply turn on the television and consider what I saw. Through my observations, He reminded me that despite the outward applause and accolades, many of such persons who decide this route of success live unfulfilled lives replete with insecurity and discontentment. This is because they choose their pursuits based upon that which they desire to *get*. However, by design, God wired us to yearn for the fulfillment of that which He seeded in us to *give*.

As I mulled over this new metric of evaluating one's life performance, I started to question whether I even knew the nature of my God-given seeds or the attributes of my "garden." However, God soon began to bring to mind those things that I do with conviction and fervor; those things for which I expend significant energy and effort to be excellent (without having to be paid to do so). These passions, I determined, were indeed my seeds. My thoughts were then directed to those events and circumstances in my life where I prevailed as an overcomer; those instances where rather than buckling under, I buckled down and stayed in the trenches. These experiences I came to realize made up the soil content of my garden. In fact, God reminded me that in the physical realm, animal manure is often used to fertilize the garden soil. (Yes, animal excrement and waste.) In the spiritual realm, we call this type of matter crises, trials and tribulations. Ha! Ultimately, from this garden, God revealed I would offer my unique contributions; that is, yield fruit of my own kind.

And so as I jotted down these thoughts that weekend before Christmas, and considered my journey thus far, I began to give God some serious praise. I was shouting and hollering all over the house. On this occasion, though, it was not because of my surgery success, but because of my fruit increase. I realized that God was simply fertilizing my garden's soil.

CHAPTER 6

"And God said, Let there be lights in the firmament of the heaven to divide the day from the night; and let them be for signs, and for seasons, and for days, and years: And let them be for lights in the firmament of the heaven to give light upon the earth: and it was so. And God made two great lights; the greater light to rule the day, and the lesser light to rule the night: He made the stars also. And God set them in the firmament of the heaven to give light upon the earth, And to rule over the day and over the night, and to divide the light from the darkness: and God saw that it was good. And the evening and the morning were the fourth day." Genesis 1: 14-19

Earthly seasons transition from one to the other without fail, but do we transition through our seasons equally as well?

From: Cynthia
Sent: Mon 01/08/2007 3:36 PM
To: Prayer Sisters
Subject: WOW!

Okay, here goes——Oh, my God! How blessed it was Saturday night! I was truly the recipient of your adherence to Paul's instructions that, "Each of you should look not only to your own interests, but also to the interests of others." (Phil. 2:4) I really don't know what to say...Well, let me try:

First, thank you, Lord for sitting in the presence of us Saturday. Thank you for anointing every act and deed that night from the soul-stirring prayer of Sister Tatum (did she not ring Heaven's doorbell Saturday?!) to the inspirational words, scriptures, and prayer sent up by my aunt, Elder Dee; from the loving words and scriptures offered by my mother to the songs of the female members of Heartspeak, the Canaan Praise Team, Phoebe Lenear, and Natalie Hamler, the presentations, and the many words of encouragement of all who were there that night.

Thank you, planning committee~ Tiffany, Larine, Joyce, Sheila, Sheena, Jayna, Jean, Carla, Lynn, and Allison~ for your incredible unselfishness in effort, time, AND money in creating such a sweet aroma for fellowship and celebration. Y'all are something else! My mom was ever so correct in saying that while this event was for me, it was not about me, but about Jesus who is working a great work in ALL of us.

Thank you, my dear sister friends, for the gifts (REALLY, y'all know I was not expecting that!). Your gifts and sentiments told me one thing, though. Clearly, you want me to relax, meditate, and rest in the Lord, and as many of you stated Saturday night, let the physical realm catch up with the spiritual realm which clearly speaks my VICTORY over this. I truly appreciate your gifts of beautiful candles, scents, inspirational books, stuffed animals, gift cards, etc. to get me there. Oh, and the pink boxing gloves, and the sling-shot (representing David's triumph over the giant Goliath and my soon triumph over cancer), and the autographed framed photo, and the personal letters——WOW, WOW, and WOW! Y'all are so awesome!

Thank you, also, dear sisters who were not able to make it, but were there in spirit celebrating. I do not take it lightly your prayers and spiritual support.

My first chemo date has been set for Friday, Jan. 19th (you know I had them schedule it after the Stellar Awards event this weekend~ ha!!~ I want to make sure that I am at the fullest cuteness that I can be for hubby! *smile*).

I am still not certain as to what my chemo treatment will entail yet (I am being considered for a clinical trial), but will let you know more specifics as soon as I get word back (i.e., time, schedule, etc.). For right now, I do want you to please pray that the treatment plan that is best for me is the clinical trial that I am selected to participate in. Talk to you soon...

Love,
Cynthia

From: Cynthia
Sent: Wed 01/17/2007 10:57 PM
To: Prayer Sisters
Subject: Round 5: For we wrestle not against flesh and blood...

My Praying Sisters,

I pray this message finds you well. I had an incredible time in Nashville this weekend at the Stellar Awards with hubby, Kevin. While he did not win (an unknown pianist by the name of Ramsey Lewis won ~*HA* ~ y'all, he's world-renowned), it WAS a stellar experience. We did the red carpet, interviews, and the whole nine yards!

Now, as I told you in my earlier email, my first chemo date has been set for this Friday, Jan. 19th. Today I found out that it will be at 9:00am (duration: 3-4 hrs). Also, as I earlier mentioned, I am participating in a clinical trial and today found out that I will be participating in a trial that requires only four (4) chemo treatments (one treatment every two weeks) for the next 8 weeks. This is a blessing, everyone—for my situation, I *could* have been doing the standard treatment which would have required 8 treatments (one treatment every 3 weeks) for a total of 24 weeks— HALLELUJAH! My remaining scheduled chemo dates are:

> Friday, Feb. 2~ 9am
> Friday, Feb. 16~ 9am
> Friday, Mar. 2~ 9am

A month following the chemo treatments, I will then begin radiation for another 5-6 weeks. So if I did my calculations correctly, I should be done with everything around mid-May. Hey, hey, hey! So here are my prayer requests this go around (the biggest issues with chemo is its potentially devastating side effects and future health risks):

1) The chemo treatment plan that I will be undergoing will be sufficient to cure me of all cancer FOREVER.
2) God will cover and protect all of my organs from any toxicity during my entire chemo and radiation process.
3) During the administration of my chemo treatments, God will guide the hands (and hearts) of the nurses who will be administering my treatment via IV.
4) I will experience NO, AND I MEAN ABSOLUTELY NO ill side effects and health risks of any sort (in the present or during my lifetime) resulting from my chemo treatment and radiation process.
5) God will strengthen my immune system throughout the chemo process so that I will stay in good health the entire time.

6) My mind will stay on Jesus and VICTORY (particularly during the 3-4 hr. process for each chemo treatment).

7) Those who surround me will only speak life and victory over this event to and for me.

8) God will continue to give me and my family peace during this event.

9) My boys will continue to not be in any way ill affected by this process.

10) I become the better and stronger physically, spiritually, and emotionally for going through this.

12) I will represent God well.

13) And foremost, God gets the total glory!

Until my next VICTORY progress report...

Love,
Cynthia

P.S. Thank you, Sister Tatum, for sharing the following scripture with me. It surely has been of great encouragement to me lately. "....Fear not: for I have redeemed thee, I have called thee by thy name; thou art mine. When thou passest through the waters, I will be with thee; and through the rivers, they shall not overflow thee: when thou walkest through the fire, thou shalt not be burned; neither shall the flame kindle upon thee." (Isaiah 43:1-2)

Over the years, my girlfriends and I have often joked about how fragile our men folks can be when dealing with some things in life. Physical pain and illness? Please pass the pacifier. Disappointments and defeat? Is there a psychologist in the house?! Life changes? Lord, help us! (Ha!) However, I must confide that as I prepared for the most intimidating round of my battle (chemotherapy), I revisited an occasion where I witnessed the greatest display of dignity and courage I had ever seen. It took place during the most difficult of life transitions, and the central character was, in fact, a *man*; specifically, my late father-in-law and Kevin's dad, Hubert Turner.

As I reflected upon memories of Mr. Turner's extraordinary poise and selflessness amid his darkest hour, they reminded me how strong and beautiful the human spirit can be, even in one's valley season. Moreover, his remarkable example recapped for me what it really means to live in the moment and let God handle the rest. Subsequently, not only was I able to go to bed at my toughest hour, I threw myself a praise party before going! (Thanks to the suggestion of another amazing *man* in my life—my father.) What follows is my account of this small but powerful chapter of his story.

Grace

I met Mr. Turner a few weeks after Kevin and I began seeing each other in the fall of '94. I was in the last year of my doctoral program at the Ohio State University in Columbus, OH, and was just beginning to seriously get to know Kevin. A native of Columbus, Kevin was an accomplished jazz guitarist and music educator. He was well-respected and admired in his community for his gifted musicianship. I had seen him on a number of occasions performing at various musical venues around town, but formally met him at New Salem Missionary Baptist Church (Pastor Keith Troy) where he and I were both members. At the time, I was involved in

New Salem's music ministry as the choir director of the youth and college choirs. Kevin played periodically with one of the other choirs in the church. While I often saw him at church, I was unaware that he had been checking me out (*smile*). Moreover, I would later find out that after sharing his interest with his close musician friend (who just happened to play for the choirs I directed), they quietly orchestrated his entrance into the band, and he soon became my bass guitarist. However, after a few months of playing a supporting role in my music ministry, he made it clear that he was vying for a leading role in my heart.

And you guessed correctly, he won.

Anyhow, shortly after Kevin and I began dating, he shared with me that his dad had recently been diagnosed with terminal lung cancer. I remember asking Kevin how his dad responded when he first received news of his cancer. Kevin said that his father turned to him at the doctor's office and stated matter-of-factly, "That's what happens when you smoke cigarettes."

Kevin indicated that his father mentioned little else about his feelings concerning his diagnosis after this. He pointed out, however, that this was not surprising. While Mr. Turner had quit smoking some twenty-five years before, Kevin noted that his dad was not one to make excuses for himself. Even when Kevin's mom passed away when he was nine, Mr. Turner fully took on the responsibility of caring for him and his two older siblings without hesitation. Thus, although I had yet to meet Kevin's dad, I knew that he was a giant of a man, like my father and grandfather. I did not realize, however, how literal this was the case until I met him for the first time.

It was a weekday morning and Mr. Turner had an appointment for radiation therapy. Kevin generally took his dad back and forth to the hospital for his treatments, and on this day I decided to accompany him. Shortly after pulling up to the front of Mr. Turner's small single-level home, the front door of the house opened to reveal the broad outline of a male figure. I then saw a silver-and-grey-peppered head covered by a wool cap dip under the top of the door frame as the towering build of an older gentleman suddenly overwhelmed the front porch.

Noticing the curious expression on my face, Kevin confirmed, "Yeah, that's my dad."

Whoa! Mr. Turner was all of 6' 5" in height. His legs had to account for nearly 5 feet of his height, I promise. At once, I climbed to the back seat of the car recognizing the need for the additional room that the front seat would provide for his dad's tall frame. Mr. Turner opened the car door and gracefully folded his long limbs into the small interior of Kevin's Toyota Corolla. His head grazed the roof's lining. Upon closing the door, he looked over at Kevin and said with a big, booming voice, "Hey!"

I could immediately tell from the tone of his greeting that he was a very pleasant fellow.

"Hey dad, this is Cindy," Kevin answered as he nodded his head back in my direction and smiled at me in his rear view mirror.

His dad turned his head towards me, gave me a quick hand wave, and said warmly, "Hey Cindy, nice to meet you."

"Nice to meet you too," I replied. Kevin had now begun making his way out of his dad's neighborhood onto the main thoroughfare.

"I hear that you are working on your doctorate degree," his dad then said, slightly leaning his head back to let me know that he was talking to me.

"Yes, I am working on my doctorate in accounting," I answered. I again made eye contact with Kevin in his rear view mirror. He had already told his dad about me!

"Um-hm…that's good," Mr. Turner responded as if impressed. "Can't be many that look like you in that field, can there," he said.

"No, you're right," I replied.

"Well, hang in there," he commented.

And that was my introduction to Mr. Turner. For the remainder of the car ride, I sat quietly as he proceeded to give Kevin an update on his favorite subject during that time—the O.J. Simpson murder case.

Over the next year, as Kevin and I became more serious, Mr. Turner's health worsened. The cancer had started showing its ugly effects, and the chemotherapy and radiation treatments had taken their toll. Nevertheless, none of this stopped my father-in-law from embracing every moment. In November of '95, he married his long-time girlfriend, Ms. Shirley Bowser, and a few weeks later, he trekked 15 hours by car to my hometown of Portsmouth, VA to see Kevin and I marry. By this time, he was a thinner and weaker frame of the man I had first met. He had lost most of his hair to chemotherapy, and was dependent on a mobile oxygen tank to help him breathe. Yet, with an oxygen tank by his side and all, he proudly delivered the Turner family welcome to me at our reception. Hm.

After our wedding, both Kevin and I left for Champaign, IL where I was now working and he was to begin graduate school. (In August of that year, I left Ohio State University with all but my dissertation completed (ABD) for an assistant professor position in the department of accountancy at the University of Illinois at Urbana-Champaign.) I urged Kevin to stay in Columbus near his father for awhile after we married, but he responded that his dad wouldn't have it. Specifically, he said that his dad told him, "Go and be with your wife. I will call you when it's time for you to come home." Hm.

Over the next few months, Kevin went through a mourning period of sorts. He struggled tremendously with what was taking place, and I really don't know how much help, if any, I was to him during this time. Kia, his teenage daughter from a previous relationship, was living with us, and that kept us pretty busy. (A teenage daughter in the house? Whew!) However, the anticipation of the now accepted inevitable was emotionally gnawing away at him, and all I could do was pray.

We got the phone call some time during the first week of March of '96. Mr. Turner told Kevin that it was time to come home.

I remember this so vividly because we were planning to return to Columbus the following week for my graduation anyhow. We had determined months earlier that the date of my graduation fell during the week of spring break for the University of Illinois. Hence, Kevin and I had already intended to spend the week with his dad. But not like this.

As we traveled to Columbus, my thoughts wandered back to an audition for a play that I had tried out for while in graduate school there. The audition required that I imagine that I was watching television when the winning lottery numbers were being revealed. I was to act out a scene in which I learned that I had the winning ticket. I was to also include in this scene my response to the subsequent event of the phone ringing and the voice on the other end telling me that my mom had just died. Boy, did I belly-flop on that audition! I decided then and there that I'd better stick with my current career path. Video footage of that audition is blackmail material for sure. Ha! Seriously, though, those range of emotions I had never experienced. So I couldn't tap into something I had never felt. That was soon to change.

We arrived late that Sunday evening.

"Kevin, your dad needs to go to the hospital, but I can't get him to go," Ms. Shirley said when we stepped inside the house. "He is not eating, and is in a lot of pain. His feet are terribly swollen and I can hardly get him out of the bed."

"Kevin, is that you?" I heard his dad say from the bedroom.

"Yeah, it's me," Kevin replied.

We walked back to Mr. Turner's bedroom to find him slumped over on the side of his bed. Unable to lift his head, he asked, "Is that Cindy with you?"

I replied, "Yes, it's me."

"Good," he answered. "I just wanted to make sure that Kevin brought the right woman home with him." Hm.

With his head still bowed, he continued, "Your big day is coming up on Friday, isn't it?"

At this point, all I could speak were one-word sentences. "Yes."

He motioned to Kevin, "Kevin, get me my wallet off the dresser."

Kevin brought his wallet over to him.

With his head still bowed, Mr. Turner fumbled through his wallet, pulled out a credit card and gave it to Kevin. "I want you to take my credit card, and tomorrow go get Cindy something for her graduation for me. Maybe a briefcase or something. Make it real nice."

Okay, dad," Kevin replied.

Hm. I was now without words.

Shortly thereafter, Mr. Turner agreed to go to the hospital. Too weak to walk, he had to be taken by the ambulance.

We did not stay with Mr. Turner at the hospital the first night. But that was the first and last time to happen. The following day, Mr. Turner told us that the nurses had been mean to him during the night, and he didn't want us to leave him alone with them anymore. Further, later that same day, the doctors had determined that the cancer had started to spread to some of his surrounding organs as well as to his brain. They said that he had only days. Consequently, he was moved to the hospice floor. And that's where we, too, set up our abode.

Thursday came, and my parents and sister arrived in town for my graduation. At this point, I was emotionally numb. My family and friends had planned a big party for me that Friday after graduation, but I could not fathom celebrating *anything*. Really, I did not even want to go to my graduation for fear of him passing away before we returned. However, I knew that no one would allow me to consider this option.

That Friday morning, Kevin took me back to his dad's house so that I could get dressed for graduation. On our ride to the house, I shared with Kevin my wish for him to go back to the hospital to be with his father. Mr. Turner's breathing had become increasingly labored over the night, and I told him that I didn't believe that he or I could handle the idea of him not being there in his dad's last moments. He agreed.

As we entered his dad's house for the first time in a few days, guess what we found sprawled from one end of the ceiling to the other? A banner that read, "Congratulations, Dr. Cynthia Turner!"

Emotionally, this was just too much. I broke down and cried. How could Mr. Turner and his family be thinking of me in such a time like this? My God. Hm.

After finally getting myself together, I met up with my family and sent Kevin back to the hospital. When we arrived on campus, my parents tried their best to encourage me. However, it was clear that I did not want to be there.

As I found my place in line and prepared myself to march in, I heard a familiar voice. It was Kevin.

"What are you doing hear?!" I exclaimed.

"My family wouldn't let me stay," Kevin replied.

"What?!"

"My sister told me to go and be with you. She promised to call when it was time."

I cried. Again. Hm.

The rest of that day was a blur to me. I was too busy praying that God would sustain Kevin's father life until Kevin got back. I vaguely remember hearing my name and crossing the stage. I faintly recall dinner afterwards with my family and friends. And I missed Kevin's cue at dinner when he told me that he would be back. He never did.

After dinner, I went to the hospital, but I wasn't allowed to go up to Mr. Turner's room. Puzzled, I called back to the house, and Kevin answered.

"Why are you and the family there?" I asked.

"Dad passed a little while ago," Kevin responded.

"Oh, Kevin, why didn't you tell me?"

"Because you didn't need to know, Cindy. This was supposed to be your day," he replied. Hm.

"Well, were you able to see him before he passed?" I asked holding my breath.

"Yes," he said.

I sighed, "Thank You, God."

"Are you okay?" I then asked.

"Yes, I'm good."

He continued, "All the family was there when he passed. Dad's breathing was really hard and his eyes were closed when I got to the room. I went around to his bedside, and my sister told him that I was there. He opened his eyes momentarily and looked at me and my sister. A tear fell down his face and then he took one last deep breath. I mean, it was like it was deliberate." Kevin paused.

"Cindy, it was as if dad had made his peace, but had held on long enough to make certain that my sister and I were there and okay." Kevin paused once more and chuckled.

"Yeah, that's just like dad—looking out for us kids until the end."

I cried. Again. Hm. This *must* be what Paul refers to as "the peace of God which passeth all understanding" (Philippians 4:7).

So the night before my first healing (chemo) treatment, I thanked God for the time He had afforded me to come to know Kevin's father. I thanked God for allowing me to bear witness to Mr. Turner's extraordinary example of grace in difficult transition. I then asked Him for a spiritual dose of what my father-in-law had, and went to bed.

(Okay, for all of you who have been keeping up—God skipped day 5 of His Creation with me initially during this journey. He can do that, you know! He takes me back to it in chapter nine, though. So hold tight. Continuing…)

CHAPTER 7

"And God said, Let the earth bring forth the living creature after his kind, cattle, and creeping thing, and beast of the earth after his kind: and it was so. And God made the beast of the earth after his kind, and cattle after their kind, and every thing that creepeth upon the earth after his kind: and God saw that it was good. And God said, Let us make man in our image, after our likeness: and let them have dominion over the fish of the sea, and over the fowl of the air, and over the cattle, and over all the earth, and over every creeping thing that creepeth upon the earth. So God created man in his own image, in the image of God created He him; male and female created He them. And God blessed them, and God said unto them, Be fruitful, and multiply, and replenish the earth, and subdue: and have dominion over the fish of the sea, and over the fowl of the air, and over every living thing that moveth upon the earth."
Genesis 1: 24-28

If we knew the power that we possessed, fear would be rendered powerless.

From: Cynthia
Sent: Fri 01/19/2007 9:34 PM
To: Prayer Sisters
Subject: RE: Round 5: For we wrestle not against flesh and blood...

You all have REALLY been praying, huh? Okay, first, though, my fault. I know I was supposed to be responsible and email you all immediately. I wanted to give myself a little time to see, but all I can say right now is "magnify the Lord with me..."

It started off slowly (4 very uncomfortable needle pricks (and three different nurses) before they could find a good vein), but then I realized. Even though we (Kevin, mom, and I) had prayed and read scripture before things got started, it was time to pray incessantly. Thus, I begin to have Kevin read scriptures aloud while the nurse prepared the medicine to be administered in my IV. Then, as the nurse began to pump the medicine in my IV, I just started praising God! In fact, my medicine is red, so I began praising God for how it reminded me of how He had washed my filthy sins away with His blood 2000 years ago. And I then began thanking Him for how He was now washing that filthy cancer right out of my body!! 4-1/2 hours later, I came out a little light-headed (Kevin and mom said I was saying all kind of silly things *smile* ~most medicine often do that to me); but no nausea, no vomiting, and I have eaten two full meals since. Hallelujah!

I am still a bit light-headed and a little fatigued, but it may be simply because of my restless 6 hours of sleep last night. What I do know, though, is that prayer does work. And YOUR prayers mean everything.

I know that I have just started this leg of the battle, and there is much more of this journey to go, but I celebrate in knowing how God showed up on THIS day. Even all of the nurses who entered that room felt compelled to share their faith's journey with us~ that's how much Jesus was in there.

Now, y'all keep praying. They ALLEGE that the first 3 days of each treatment are the worst. We are praying against that. NO NAUSEA, NO VOMITING, AND NO ILL SIDE EFFECTS OF ANY SORT! They also say that with the medication that I am on, I will most likely lose my hair in the next week or two. So IF God chooses to allow this and I have to do the wig thing, I got that covered, and those of you in town, better say I look cute (LOL)! (I may try some things...)

Will keep you posted as the days go by. But know that I feel SO blessed to have you as my praying sisters!

Love,
Cynthia

From: Cynthia
Sent: Sat 01/20/2007 8:17 PM
To: Prayer Sisters
Subject: RE(2): Round 5: For we wrestle not against flesh and blood...

Day 2 (of supposedly the worst 3 days of each treatment):

Okay, I had to share this with you. I had to go in today to get a shot of Neulasta (to boost my immune system; chemo treatments depress your immune system which makes you very susceptible to infections). Anyhow, the nurse who was administering the medication asked me if this was my first time taking this shot, and I said, "yes." Then she proceeded to tell me how these shots were very painful and would really burn. I mean, y'all, she repeated this more than once and emphasized that while she was going to administer it very slowly, still expect it to burn alot.

Now, come on. My initial thought was why did she tell me that? Especially when I knew that I had to take these shots after the next three treatments as well...Anyways, she then says, "Are you ready?" At that point, I begin mentally repeating to myself, "Cynthia doesn't do burns, and God will not give me any more than I can bear." I heard Kevin muttering something under his breath as well, but I wouldn't find out until later exactly what he was mumbling~"Cynthia will not feel a thing." (Sisters, God has really been speaking to me (via His Word, and some awesome books and tapes) regarding the power of one's mind. And all who really know me, know that I am EXTREMELY dramatic and emotional when it comes to EVEN REMOTE possible pain. So for me to even mentally respond with assuredness was a MIRACLE!

Well, as that needle entered the back of my arm, can I tell you that not only did I not feel a burning sensation of any sort, but I did not even feel the needle enter my arm! The only reason I knew that she was administering the shot was because she kept asking, "Are you doing okay?" every few seconds. I kept looking for the burning to begin, but the next thing I know, she was saying, "All done." Actually, I think she was so taken aback by my non-response that she started saying, "You know, I've been told that when you administer it slowly, it reduces the burning, so just tell the nurse who administers it next time to do it slowly it as well."

My answer: God IS faithful. *All the Time*

"Now this is the confidence (notice it doesn't say "doubt") we have in Him, that if we ask anything according to His Will (and His Word is His Will), He hears us. And if we know that He hears us, whatever we ask, we know that we have the petitions that we have asked of Him." (I John 5:14-15)

We serve such a MIGHTY God! HALLELUJAH!

From: Cynthia
Sent: Tue 01/23/2007 2:07 PM
To: Prayer Sisters
Subject: RE(3): Round 5: For we wrestle not against flesh and blood...

Okay, I promise, very short...I went in today to have a groshong catheter (a silicon tube) implanted in my chest so that I will not have any repeat episodes of my earlier problematic IV needle issues. Specifically, this will allow the medical staff to do my lab work and administer the treatments through this tube. But, of course, the assisting nurse had to share with me the particulars of the procedure and all of the potential problems. (I will not even begin to tell you what she shared. Just suffice to know that Kevin asked me afterwards, "Are you sure you want to do this?")

Well, there was no sedation for this procedure, and the only medication that was used was the novacaine that was externally administered at the two areas where the doctor inserted the tube and where the tube was to come out...I started praying, of course. The doctor overheard me and asked me what I was saying. "Just praying for God's guidance over your hands and this procedure," I replied. He responded, "Well, I can always use more help."

Despite the doctor's warning of probable burning and discomfort as he pushed the catheter through (with a knitting needle, mind you), I had NO PAIN, NO BURNING, AND NO DISCOMFORT. Afterwards, the nurse said to me, "You were such a great patient. You did not move at all and did so well." I responded, "I just made certain that the Master Physician was looking on."

She then replied, "There is really something to believing in God isn't it?" Why did she say that? I began with, "Can I tell you more?"

From: Cynthia
Sent: Thu 02/ 01/2007 3:04 PM
To: Prayer Sisters
Subject: Round 6: For we wrestle not against flesh and blood...

My Praying Sisterfriends,

God is good all the time, and all the time... I just left the doctor's office for my first check-up since chemo. Results so far:

- White blood count~ excellent (reflects condition of immune system)
- Platelet count~ excellent (reflects condition of immune system)
- hair~ still got it for now (*smile*; don't know what to do with it though~ can't get my routine perm!)
- nausea/vomiting~ none
- mouth sores~ none

Yes, yes, and yes. God is faithful and does answer prayers! The only concern at the moment is that my red blood count is low (I am a bit anemic). So, as I go in tomorrow for my second chemo treatment, I ask that you please pray for the following (much of the same):

1) The chemo treatment plan that I will be undergoing will be sufficient to cure me of all cancer FOREVER.
2) God will continue to cover and protect all of my organs from any toxicity during my entire chemo and radiation process.
3) I will continue to experience NO, AND I MEAN ABSOLUTELY NO ill side effects and health risks of any sort (in the present or during my lifetime) resulting from my chemo treatment and radiation process.
4) God will continue to strengthen my immune system throughout the chemo process so that I will stay in good health the entire time (good white blood cell count and platelet count).

5) God will build my red blood count to its appropriate levels for the remainder of my treatment.

6) My mind will stay on Jesus and VICTORY (particularly during the 3-4 hr. process for each chemo treatment).

7) Those who surround me will only speak life and victory over this event to and for me.

8) God will continue to give me and my family peace during this event.

9) My boys will continue to not be in any way ill affected by this process.

10) I become the better and stronger physically, spiritually, and emotionally for going through this.

11) I will represent God well.

12) And foremost, God gets the total glory!

Until my next VICTORY progress report...

Love,
Cynthia

"....Fear not: for I have redeemed thee, I have called thee by thy name; thou art mine. When thou passest through the waters, I will be with thee; and through the rivers, they shall not overflow thee: when thou walkest through the fire, thou shalt not be burned; neither shall the flame kindle upon thee...." (Isaiah 43:1-2)

From: Cynthia
Sent: Tue 02/06/2007 3:48 PM
To: Prayer Sisters
Subject: RE: Round 6: For we wrestle not against flesh and blood...

My Beautiful Praying Sister Warriors,

Thank you for your unceasing prayers. God is good ALL of the time. Days 2 and 3 since my last *healing* treatment have proved to be the toughest days yet, but at worst, it has been a battle with fatigue and the metal-mouth taste. God didn't say that this was going to be a smooth ride all the way, but He did promise that

He would ride along with me. Consequently, I have yet to miss a meal (regardless of how it has tasted), and I still have not experienced any vomiting, mouth sores, etc. Praise Him! I am starting to shed some hair now, but I have already made preparation for this. My boys have finally given me the green light on the wig selection (*smile*), so I am good to go there. (We had a couple of Elvis Presley impersonation moments during this selection process, though—ha!)

I am already half-way through this part of the process (this is the 2nd of 4 treatments), can you believe it? And I promise you, if fatigue, metal-mouth, and short-term hair loss are all that I must face for another 6-12 weeks to add 60+ years to my life, so be it. I will simply be a sleeping, ginger-drinking, hat-, scarf-, and wig-wearing sister on fire for the Lord for the time being!

Please continue to hold me and my family's strength and endurance up in prayer and I will further update you regarding my VICTORY progress shortly.

Love,
Cynthia

"They that wait upon the Lord SHALL renew their strength, they SHALL mount up with wings as of eagles, they SHALL run and not be weary and they SHALL walk and not faint!" (Isaiah 40:31)

From: Cynthia
Sent: Fri 02/ 09/2007 11:41 AM
To: Prayer Sisters
Subject: RE(2): Round 6: For we wrestle not against flesh and blood...

I surely know who to hook up with to get prayer through. Thank you, sisters! I feel SO much better today. Actually, I started feeling much better Wednesday evening. Again, God is ALL that! Funny thing, as I mentioned to you earlier, I started shedding my hair this week. So, I decided to go ahead Wednesday evening and let my hair go. Of course, I gave my hubby, Kevin, the honors. Now, Kevin has been bald for some time now, so he should be an old pro, right? Well, I forgot that he uses Bic razors for his head, and I was not ready to go that route immediately. At least, let the process be gradual. So we started with clippers first.

Kevin pulls out some clippers he has had probably since before we were married (we've been married for 11 years now). He blows the dust off the clippers first~ bad sign already. He plugs the clippers in and turns the clippers on.

ARRRGGGHHHHHH!!!!!! ARRRGGGHHHHHH!!!!!! ARRRGGGHHHHHH!!!!!!

Have you ever ridden by a construction site when workers are drilling into cement? Well, imagine that sound in my small kitchen coming from these clippers. The sound itself nearly scared the hair off my head! Lord knows, this was NOT helping. Poor sweetheart, Kevin, with his screwdriver, just busily working on the clippers. Anyhow, he finally gets the sound to a tolerable noise level.

"Are you ready?" he asks. I simply said, "Jesus."

Bzzzzzzzz. And off my hair went. Women, what an experience! I didn't know what to feel~ fear and anxiousness or liberation and peace! I wouldn't even look. Leave it, though, to God to move my husband to say just the right thing with so much convictedness, "Wow, girl, you look FINE!"

"Do I really?" I responded. So I finally looked.

God is just SO good! My perfectly round shaped head was peeking back at me reminding me how perfect God is! It reminded me of the scripture, "I am fearfully and wonderfully made" (Psalm 139:14). I looked again. I saw my two boys, Julien and Justen, in the mirror...amazing...

However, by that time, Kevin thought that perhaps I needed a little more professional assistance, and my beautiful hair stylist and angel, Christina, trudged through the late night hour AND snow to attend to me. We ALL grew up Wednesday night.

By yesterday (Thursday), it became clear that the short crop hairdo would not work. Patches had begun to fall out every-where I scratched. Like I shared with my mom and sisters, by yesterday evening, I looked liked a little Ethiopian boy with a bad case of ringworm (LOL). Every time I passed by the mirror, I would say to myself, "poor thing!" (HA!) Hence, last night, I granted my husband the rights to take me down to a buzz and so I am now a full-fledged G.I. Jane, y'all, and proud!

Just wanted you to know that I am doing well and to God be the glory! Again, thank you for your prayers, and I will keep you posted.

Love,
Cynthia

From: Cynthia
Sent: Mon 02/12/2007 8:04 PM
To: Prayer Sisters
Subject: Round 7: For we wrestle not against flesh and blood...

Well, spirit-filled women, we are fast approaching healing treatment # 3 (of 4) already. I am doing really well. Really, after one can get past the first few days, you can go on with daily activities within reason. I am told, though, that as the treatments progress, the chronic fatigue, metal-mouth, and the overall feeling of blah tends to persist longer and longer, so I want to get a jumpstart on my prayer requests this go around. So here they are:

1) *The chemo treatment plan that I will be undergoing will be sufficient to cure me of all cancer FOREVER.*

2) *God will continue to cover and protect all of my organs from any toxicity during my entire chemo and radiation process.*

3) *I will continue to experience NO, AND I MEAN ABSOLUTELY NO ill side effects and health risks of any sort (in the present or during my lifetime) resulting from my chemo treatment and radiation process.*

4) *God will continue to strengthen my immune system throughout the chemo process so that I will stay in good health the entire time (good white blood cell count and platelet count); AND folks will be sensitive enough to not come around me when they are ill.*

5) *God will minimize the fatigue, nausea, metal-mouth, and feelings of blah during the first week following the remaining healing treatments.*

6) *God will build my red blood count to its appropriate levels for the remainder of my treatment.*

7) *My mind will stay on Jesus and VICTORY (particularly during the 3-4 hr. process for each chemo treatment).*

8) *Those who surround me will only speak life and victory over this event to and for me.*

9) *God will continue to give me and my family peace during this event.*

10) *My boys will continue to not be in any way ill affected by this process.*

11) *I become the better and stronger physically, spiritually, and emotionally for going through this.*

12) *I will represent God well.*

13) *And foremost, God gets the total glory!*

I will talk with you on the other side of healing treatment # 3.

Love,
Cynthia

P.S. When I finally let my boys see my new G.I. Jane look, my baby boy, Justen (4-1/2), looked in awe (eyes bucked wide open), paused, and said emphatically, "Mom, I want you to have your hair back." And a few minutes later after it appears he gave it a little more thought, he stated, "And keep a scarf or wig on your head until your hair grows back UP!" (I laughed so hard, y'all, I almost could not contain myself!) So not to traumatize my boys, I keep something on my head when they are around. When they are not, I let my head BREATHE in Jesus' name (LOL).

From: Cynthia
Sent: Fri 02/16/2007 10:12 PM
To: Prayer Sisters
Subject: RE(2): Round 7: For we wrestle not against flesh and blood...

Ladies,

Three down, one more to go! Isn't He good!! Please pray for my STRENGTH (no nausea, no metal mouth, minimal fatigue, minimal blah) during the next 7 days. Thank you!

Will keep you posted.

-Cynthia

From: Cynthia
Sent: Fri 02/23/2007 7:22 AM
To: Prayer Sisters
Subject: RE(3): Round 7: For we wrestle not against flesh and blood...

Hey, women! Yes, I believe I can see the finish line now...hey, hey, hey! Got a head cold that seems to not want to go away, but my strength is increasing daily. The metal mouth left me around Wednesday, and now I'm just trying to shake off the fatigue.

Next Friday, Mar. 2 (9am) is my last healing treatment date, and then we move on to radiation for 6 weeks. Will email you with my next prayer requests early next week. Until then, please continue to pray my strength and overcoming this cold.

From: Cynthia
Sent: Fri 03/02/2007 7:44 AM
To: Prayer Sisters
Subject: Round 8: For we wrestle not against flesh and blood...

Victory is mine, victory is mine, victory today is mine! 9:00am (10am EST), women, please join me in praying this:

"Lord, we know that Jesus bore our sins in His own body on the tree, that we, having died to sins, might live for righteousness—for whose stripes we were healed. And for this reason, Lord, we give thanks unto You and call upon Your name making known Your deeds among the people of how you have blessed Cynthia through this stage of her healing process. We pray, Lord, that Cynthia will seek You and Your strength: seeking Your face evermore. We pray that Cynthia will remember Your marvelous works that You have done and Your wonders. And as Cynthia begins this last healing treatment this morning, we pray that her light shall break forth like the morning, her healing shall spring forth speedily, and the glory of You will be her rear guard! In your precious Son, Jesus' name, AMEN.

-(Taken from 1 Pet. 2:24; Psalm 105:4,5; Isaiah 58:8)

Thank you, sisters, and I will talk to you on the other side.

Love you,
Cynthia

Clearly God intended for us to have dominion and power over all things of this world. He said it! "Let them (man and woman) have dominion over the fish of the sea, and over the fowl of the air, and over the cattle, and over all the earth, and over every creeping thing that creepeth upon the earth"

(Genesis 1:26). Still, at the beginning of the chemo process (before the miraculous events detailed in the previous emails), I questioned did I get the point—did I *really* get the intended point of this day of Creation. And you know why? Because despite going to bed at peace the night before my first chemo session, I awoke during the wee hours of that morning— scared silly!

Yes, somewhere between 4 and 6am that morning, I found myself pulling out the sword of the Spirit, the Word (see Ephesians 6:17), trying to restore some calm. Interestingly, as I scoured God's Word during those pre-dawn hours, He directed me back to the scripture passage concerning Adam's fall (see Genesis 3). And it was in my re-examination of this text that I soon discovered something I had not seen before. Ultimately, this something helped me to stay in the trenches for the morning skirmish, and fortified my position for the remaining ones that followed. Now, we all know Adam's story, don't we?

Naked

Satan, disguised as a crafty serpent, approached Eve and enticed her to eat of the tree of knowledge. Eve, in turn, convinced Adam to do the same, and the scriptures say that their eyes were opened, and they realized that they were naked (Genesis 3:7). Subsequently, Adam and Eve covered themselves and went into hiding because they were afraid (Genesis 3:8-10).

Let me stop here.

On that morning, when I got to this point, I considered again the last detail—when they realized that they were naked, they became afraid.

Being then lead, I grabbed my high school thesaurus[1] to look up other synonyms for the word, "naked." The following synonyms were provided: "exposed," "uncovered," "visible," "undisguised," "vulnerable."

Still being prompted, I pulled out my dictionary and looked up the definition of the synonym that stood out to me— "vulnerable." The definition read, "to be open to attack."

I went back to the passage and replaced the word, "naked," so that it now read:

> "And the Lord God called unto Adam and said unto him, Where art thou? And he said, I heard thy voice in the garden, and I was afraid, because I was *open to attack*; and I hid myself. And (God) said, who told thee that thou was *open to attack*?" (Genesis 3:9-11).

When I read those words aloud, I broke down and sobbed. It was as if God was asking me that very question— "Yes, Cynthia, who told you that you were open to attack? Do you not know my promises of protection?"

I then took out my Rhodes' (2003) book of Bible promises[2] and thumbed through the pages until I got to the section concerning God's protection. I began to speak the following:

> "He will cover you with His feathers, and under His wings you will find refuge; His faithfulness will be your shield and rampart. You will not fear the terror of night, nor the arrow that flies by day; nor the pestilence that stalks in the darkness, nor the plague that destroys at midday." (Psalm 91:4-6, NIV)

> "Because he loves me," says the Lord, "I will rescue him; I will protect him, for he acknowledges my name." (Psalm 91:14, NIV)

> "The Lord loves the just and will not forsake his faithful ones. They will be protected forever, but the offspring of the wicked will be cut off." (Psalm 37:28, NIV)

> "The Lord is faithful, and He will strengthen and protect you from the evil one." (2 Thessalonians 3:3, NIV)

> "If you make the Most High your dwelling—even the Lord, who is my refuge—then no harm will befall you, no disaster will come near your tent." (Psalm 91:9-10, NIV)

> "The Lord will keep you from all harm—He will watch over your life; the Lord will watch over your coming and going both now and forevermore." (Psalm 121:7-8, NIV)

As I spoke each one of these promises, I began to feel my calm returning. Whoa! I now realized why satan was considered so cunning. From the beginning of time, he knew that if he could awaken our awareness to our human vulnerabilities, he could separate us from the source which gave us *divine* authority—our Creator and our Lord.

But, in those early morning hours, God pointed out to me that He closed this divide between humanity and divinity when He wrapped His Son in flesh to walk perfectly among us over two thousand years ago. Further, God reminded me that, when His Son and our Savior, Jesus Christ, triumphed over the grave with all power, He also reclaimed our authority over this earth, giving us the right to walk in victory over every circumstance.

So as I got dressed and prepared myself for my first session, I once again thanked God for His promises of protection and my certain victory. And then right before I headed out the door, I checked to make certain I had everything—my Bible, my laptop, my water, my crackers and…yeah, my notes from that morning. I didn't want the enemy getting that close to me again. I had a victory to claim! *In Jesus name Amen*

"In all these things we are more than conquerors *through* Him that loved us." (Romans 8:37, NIV)

CHAPTER 8

*(I just had to share with you another divine movement of God done
during another of my dark moments. Revisit chapter two for the
background.)*

When you can't see your way, turn up your audio.
God may be giving directions.

From: Cynthia
Sent: Wed 03/07/2007 8:37 PM
To: Prayer Sisters
Subject: RE: Round 8: For we wrestle not against flesh and blood...

Woooooooo........................Y'all, this last one was a doozy. Thank you so much for keeping me lifted in prayer! I am completely drained and am recovering from a sinus infection (I am on antibiotics), but I AM DONE with this stage of the process~ HALLELUJAH! When I have a bit more strength I will share more, but know that I am hanging in there and God is good.

Love,
Cynthia

From: Cynthia
Sent: Wed 03/14/2007 12:00 PM
To: Prayer Sisters
Subject: RE(2): Round 8: For we wrestle not against flesh and blood...

Okay, can I testify? This is bit long. When I wrote you last Wednesday, I had no idea that I was about to face my most formidable day yet (Letha, you were right). However, on last Thursday, March 8, I had to be at the lowest point I had been throughout this process. Literally, Thursday morning when I awoke, I could barely move out of my bed. As you know, my last healing treatment was administered on Friday, Mar. 2. (Praise the Lord!) On the night of that treatment, though, it was really tough, and yet, I had no clue it would get worse. I had experienced fatigue before with the other treatments, but not of this magnitude. At best as I can explain, it is a bone-weary fatigue where you feel as if weights are placed on your extremities. What made it worse was that I was taking antibiotics that were having their own side effects, along with the fact that I had lost my sense of taste and smell because of my sinus infection, AND the absolute worse was that while my body wanted to rest, my mind didn't.

I had heard of "racing thoughts" before when speaking of mental patients. They are thoughts that just won't be quiet; they can gallop around in one's head like a carousel gone out of control. However, I had never experienced it, until that week. I would lie down, but my mind would constantly keep racing. Thus, even though my eyes were closed, it was difficult to go to sleep. In fact, from Friday, Mar. 2 to Thursday, Mar. 8, I thought I was losing it! I would wake up in the middle of the night at least 4-5 times. Every little sound would wake me. But God...

Thursday morning, I told Kevin that something had to give. I was at a breaking point. God had to show up. I had decided if things did not get any better by the afternoon, I was going to visit the doctor. I went back to bed after Kevin and the boys had left for the day, and the phone rang. Of course, I was too tired to pick up the phone. The phone had rung numerous times before on that morning, but no one had left a message. However, at 11:11am (according to the answering machine), My Aunt (Rev.) Dee (a number of you met her at my praise party) called and left a message. She was planning a conference this fall and wanted to talk to me about be one of the speakers. I heard the message while she was leaving it, and immediately, I was uplifted because it was as if God was reminding me that this experience was bigger than me. Further, it was at that moment that I could softly hear him saying to me, "How can you testify of My goodness and be a witness to those who have gone through and who will be going through this, if you don't experience a bit of what most experience throughout their ENTIRE treatment process? I've only allowed you to experience this at your last treatment."

In the meantime, I heard the customary ring on my computer indicating that I had new email messages. I decided at that point that I would get up and check my messages (I had not checked them for several days at that point). Well, lo, and behold, there is a message time-stamped 11:10am from sister, Tammy Taylor, subject titled, "RE: Cancer."

Now, you know, after having not checked my messages in days, there were a multitude of messages. However, because of the nature of the title, I was praying that that message could possibly speak to my situation. Upon opening the message and reading, I could only get three-quarters of the way through the message, before I just began praising God. Tammy had forwarded to me a message from a brother in Christ whose name is Terrence.

I had never personally met him, but I knew of him through Tammy and his wife, Jewyl (Terrence and Jewyl own Ringspirations.com, a Christian ringtone company). The message began, "Hey Tammy, thinking about sister Turner this morning and her cancer challenge. It prompted me to call a claimant back that I had spoken with a few weeks ago. She had advanced 4th stage cancer..."

He went on to share that this woman, Linda Booth, has been cancer-free since 2005 and attributed a product called Cellfood to, among other things, giving her energy throughout her treatments. Her recovery had convinced her doctor of its benefits so much so that he has allowed her to share this information with his patients as they sit in the lobby waiting to see him. Further, because of her deep belief in this the product, she is now a sales representative for the company. Terrence went on to say that he, too, was convinced that there was something to this product, and that he was willing to buy me my first bottle.

But sisters, he did not have to do any convincing, that was God speaking directly to me. God HAD shown up! I immediately called Kevin, and on his lunch break, he came and picked me up. With what remaining strength I could muster, I went with Kevin to our local natural food store, and I purchased me a bottle of Cellfood. (It's a liquid concentrate of 129 trace nutrients and electrolytes that is attributed to releasing oxygen and hydrogen to all the cells in the human body to aid the immune system and detoxify the body of toxins. You place 8 drops of this in spring water or juice 3x /day.)

I began taking the Cellfood that afternoon and by that evening, when the boys came home, I felt better. Further, I was amazed as to what was to follow—that night I slept through the entire night for the first time in seven days. And Friday, oh, Friday, when I woke up, honestly, I felt like a NEW woman. I woke Kevin up ecstatic! I could NOT believe how energetic I felt. I had not felt this way since before starting my chemo treatments. In fact, I was feeling so good that after Kevin and the boys left for the day, I got on the treadmill and vigorously walked a mile, something I had not done in weeks! And, as a consequence I then bought two more bottles of Cellfood Friday afternoon and overnighted them to my parents.

Sisters, you never know how God might use any one of us to be a blessing to someone. And, now, even though I've always had head knowledge of this, I now have heart knowledge that there are no such things as coincidences in this life. Events are either God-orchestrated or God-allowed. Thursday, March 8 was God-orchestrated for me. Thus, I thank YOU for praying for me incessantly, and I praise God that Terrence and Tammy were available and obedient to God's prodding and direction.

Isn't God something? I am just amazed how He can place me on the mind of a brother (who I have never met) to such a degree that he feels compelled to take the time to gather and share this information with my sister, who then, out of obedience, immediately passes the information along at the very moment I needed it the most. How else can you explain it? But God...

I feel like Joseph did when speaking to his brothers, "You intended to harm me, but God intended it for good to accomplish what is now being done..."(Gen. 50:20) The devil intended this condition to harm me, but God intended it for good.

I want you to know that I am doing SO, SO much better, and I am getting stronger everyday. I meet with my oncologist on April 5 for my follow-up. Please continue to pray for my strength and keep my family in prayer, and I will keep you posted.

He's awesome,
Cynthia

"And we know that ALL things work together for the good to them who love God, to them who are the called according to His purpose." Romans 8:28

---

*N*eed I say more?!

(As I mentioned in chapter 7, God shared with me insights of day 5 of His Creation a bit later in my journey. Well, this was the leg…)

CHAPTER 9

"And God said, Let the waters bring forth abundantly the moving creature that hath life, and fowl that may fly above the earth in the open firmament of heaven. And God created great whales, and every living creature that moveth, which the waters brought forth abundantly, after their kind, and every winged fowl after his kind: and God saw that it was good. And God blessed them, saying, Be fruitful, and multiply, and fill the waters in the seas, and let fowl multiply in the earth. And the evening and the morning were the fifth day." Genesis 1: 20-23

For every distinct creation God made, separate quarters to each He assigned. Since you and I share in the same earthly space, less different we must be by design. Let's start acting like it!

From: Cynthia
Sent: Wed 04/04/2007 12:58 PM
To: Prayer Sisters
Subject: Doctor's Visit Tomorrow

Hello Beautiful Sisters,

Stop worrying! (*smile*) I am doing great. My energy is excellent, and I am starting to feel like my old self. Now, how I look, that's another story. (Ha!) Would you believe that I started losing (and lost) all of my eyebrows last week? (Three weeks after my last treatment.) So in my full naturalness, I look like one of those robots from Will Smith's ,"I, Robot." In fact, I was joking with my nurse that without hair and eyebrows, this cancer thing really unites us as a people because we ALL look alike.

Anyway, the other funny part is this wig thing. You wig-wearing sisters should have forewarned me. First, no one told me that wearing a wig would be SO hot! So until my hair grows back, you won't be seeing me with wigs on unless I am going to church or somewhere special. Scarves will have to do. Also, no one told me that when you wear a synthetic wig, you can't be near hot areas. (Ha!) I was thinking I was looking cute with this shoulder-length auburn wig that I had on (yes, off black tipped with medium auburn~ T130/1B) until I took some food out of the oven. I knew I smelled something, but thought it was the food. Hush your mouth, later on, I was in the bathroom and noticed that the front of my hair looked awfully strange. Upon further investigation, lo and behold, I realized that all of the front of my wig had shriveled up from the heat of the oven!! I still have a lot to learn... I go to see my doctor for my first follow-up after my healing treatments TOMORROW (11:15am), girls! Keep me lifted and I will talk to you on the other side.

Love,
Cynthia

G rowing up, there were three things that my dad, Rev. Franklin R. Williams, expected of each of his four children in our household—respect, appreciation, and love for one another. That is, we were to show love and respect to my mom (aka, Mary P.) and him. We were to display our appreciation for that which they provided to and for us. (My dad made tremendous sacrifices during our childhood to make certain that we not only got what we needed, but what we wanted.) Finally, we were to always exhibit love for one another.

In general, I think we met dad's first two expectations with little required assistance. I believe this to be the case because my dad and mom's style of facilitation was not widely embraced by us children. Ha! (Yes, we learned at a very early age that obedience was better than sacrifice.)

However, from time to time, the "show love for one another" principle proved to be a tall order. Now, believe you me, we loved—and still do love—each other completely and unconditionally. In fact, other kids often thought twice before battling with one of us because they knew it may be costly. Yet, our "display" of love for one another was not always in view. You see, we were all quite different, and our differences, when not managed properly, would lead to conflict.

Take for example my relationship with my sister Celia. She was just a year younger than I, but by the time I was 3 or 4 years old, she and I were the same size. As a result, we were often mistaken to be twins until she shot pass me in height some time during our elementary school years. Hence, the ongoing conflict for us was concerning who was the boss. I was older, but she was taller and bigger— and had a "heavy hand." Ouch!

Then, there was my baby sister, Frances. She was four years younger. That four-year difference (which is now trivial) was *huge* to my sister Celia and me when growing up. Thus, we often struggled with the fact that Frances insisted on being included in everything that we did, and knew how to whine just long enough to get my parents to agree.

My brother, Clint, was the baby *and* the only boy in our family. And so, you likely already know what our issues were with him—he was spoiled rotten! He got almost anything he wanted, and got away with almost everything he did. (I may be exaggerating ever so slightly.) But really! At times, we would marvel at the ease in which he skated through certain situations (if we could have been as lucky). Our parents' justification? They were older and had simply grown tired by the time he was born. He was eight years younger.

Now, I readily admit that I, too, had my own set of issues. I was the first-born, and so I was the "show-off" child.

Meaning, when family and friends came around, I was usually given the green light to "show off." Thus, at the appointed time, I would try to amaze the adults with my reading skills (my parents would have me read from the encyclopedia when I was 5); or attempt to dazzle them with my dancing skills (I could do a *mean* robot); or aim to delight them with my ability to sing and play the piano. The problem was I did not know how to turn my "show" off!

Might you know of other children like that? Every time they think that you may be watching, they begin to showcase one of their talents; in every photograph taken, they find a way of putting themselves in it. Well, yep, that was me—and I believe now that child is my baby boy, Justen. Lawd.

I also suffered with severe allergies when I was young (as mentioned in earlier chapters). Consequently, I tended to make rather irritating noises during my seasonal episodes. Snorting, sniffling and scratching of the throat were my typical aural reactions. My sister Celia was the least apprecia-tive of them, and would often hurl pillows and other objects at me to show her repugnance. (Poor Julien, my oldest, I believe picked up those unfortunate traits.)

Nevertheless, despite our idiosyncrasies and differences, my siblings and I were deeply connected by our commonly shared family values and experiences. Further, we were blessed to be guided by loving parents who ensured that we always worked through our conflicts— one way or another.

Well, when I tried to make application of the fifth day of the Creation to my battle, God brought these memories to mind. And He did so while I, along with seven other patients, underwent our chemotherapy sessions at the cancer treatment center. This happened to be my last visit.

The treatment room, which was mainly circular in shape, consisted of reclining chairs that sat side-by-side around its exterior. The resulting open space took a little getting used to when I first began chemo because it allowed us as patients to easily see one another during the administration of our treatments. By this visit, though, I was quite comfortable with the setting since it often lead us to encourage each other and share in our experiences and struggles.

When I surveyed the room, I noticed that I was the youngest and the only one of color on this occasion, but most of us were bald with some degree of facial hair loss (i.e., loss of eyebrows and/or eyelashes). Six of us were women while the other two were men. The woman to my right looked like she could have been in her early fifties. Wisps of thin blonde hair peeked from under her tan baseball cap. Her thin, oval-shaped glasses contrasted against her fair complexion that was now completely void of all facial hair. She was comfortably reclined in her chair with a colorful blanket covering her. She was reading intensely a book while her medication steadily dripped from her IV bag.

To my far left, was another woman who appeared to be old enough to be my grandmother. She, too, was wrapped in a blanket that I imagined she likely crocheted herself. She was fast asleep as her medication flowed through her IV. Her husband sat dutifully by her side. To pass the time, he divided his attention between watching the flat screen television in the room and reading several magazines. Similarly, the others in the room were either watching television, reading or resting.

That day, I had on my customary session garb which included a black scarf, jeans, and a buttoned-down top. The buttoned-down top was necessary because of how my medication was now administered. As I mentioned earlier, after my first eventful session where it took the nurses four attempts to find a vein, I had a groshong catheter temporarily implanted in my chest. The nurses needed now only attach the IV line to this tube in order to administer my medication. Hence, a buttoned-down top made it convenient for them to readily access it.

I could only imagine, though, what the other patients and families thought when Kevin and I would come to these sessions. As I noted earlier, most chose to relax during this time by reading, resting or watching television; but not

Kevin and me. We had to bring our own modes of tranquility. Kevin brought his guitar (surprise!) and I brought my laptop. And while it never quite worked out that Kevin got the chance to play, I did spend much of my time writing.

In the midst of my writing on this day, God pressed me to canvass the room once again. This time, He moved me to consider the scene before me in light of those family memories upon which I had just reflected. I soon began to realize how, like my siblings, we—who were sitting in the room—were all different, and yet we were related. Only in this case, we were related by the commonly shared experience of cancer. We were all in the same fight, and our ordeals with this sickness had linked us together. As such, all other details seemed insignificant—race, age, sex, culture, socio-economic background, and the like. However, God would not let me rest with that thought.

"Are you *only* connected by this experience? Am I *not* the Father of all mankind?" I heard Him softly ask. It then dawned on me how wise indeed my dad had been in raising his children. For as I began to embrace the point that God was trying to make—we were all family members of humanity, guess what I soon determined to be God's expectations of each one of us?

Reverence (respect):
"Should you not fear me?" declares the Lord. Should you not tremble in my presence? I made the sand a boundary for the sea, and everlasting barrier it cannot cross. The waves may roll, but they cannot prevail; they may roar, but they cannot cross it." (Jeremiah 5:22, NIV)

"Who will not fear You, O Lord, and bring glory to your name? For You alone are holy: All nations will come and worship before You; for your righteous acts have been revealed." (Revelations 15:4, NIV)

Praise (appreciation):
"Give thanks to the Lord, call on his name; make known among the nations what He has done." (I Chronicles 16:8, NIV)

"Therefore, since we are receiving a kingdom that cannot be shaken, let us be thankful, and so worship God acceptably with reverence and awe, for our "God is a consuming fire." (Hebrews 12: 28-29, NIV)

Love:
"… Love the Lord your God with all your heart and with all your soul and with all your mind. This is the first and greatest commandment. And the second is like it: *Love your neighbor as yourself.*" (Matthew 22:37-39, NIV)

In the end, I concluded that, as family members of the human race, we had the very same problem that my siblings and I had growing up. We needed to work on the "show love one to another" principle. I just prayed then and there that God would not have to step in and facilitate this process in the same manner that my parents did when we were young. But then again, my dad took his principles from the Good Book.

CHAPTER 10

"And God said, Behold, I have given you every herb bearing seed, which upon the face of all the earth, and every tree, in which is the fruit of a tree yielding seed; to you it shall be meat. And to every beast of the earth and to every fowl of the air, and to every thing that creepeth upon the earth, wherein there is life, I have given every green herb for meat: and it was so. And God saw every thing that he had made, and behold, it was very good. And the evening and the morning were the sixth day." Genesis 1: 29-31

Have you tried God's Foods lately? All produce are YHVH-approved and Lord-certified. Restoration guaranteed.

From: Cynthia
Sent: Fri 04/06/2007 6:48 PM
To: Prayer Sisters
Subject: RE: Doctor's Visit

Doctor said my vitals and lab reports were EXCELLENT! (Specifically she said, "I know you likely have never had anyone to rave over your vitals before, have you? You're perfect.") More details later. Happy Easter! We serve a VICTORIOUS Savior!

-Cynthia

After having a heart attack in 1995, my grandfather, Samuel W. Pinner, decided to change his lifestyle at the tender age of 75. Prompted also by the discovery that he was overweight, diabetic and had Parkinson's Disease, my grandfather embarked upon changes in his diet and exercise regimen literally overnight. He went from eating virtually anything he liked (which included many foods seasoned with high-fat, high-sugar and high-salt) to eating only broiled, baked and boiled dishes flavored with minimal seasoning (Ms. Dash to be more specific). He changed his sedentary ways of little-to-no regular exercise to a routine that included a 5-mile brisk walk three times a week, religiously. As a result, granddad lost forty pounds in a month's time and never had to go on any medication until he was diagnosed with prostate cancer in 2006. His goal was to reach the hearty age of 100.

When I learned of my illness, I immediately thought of my grandfather and his resolve. His example became my inspiration as I sought to make similar changes in my life. And while granddad missed his mark by a few years (he died in September 2007), his resilience and strength has left an indelible impression on my life that just may serve to help me reach that age myself.

Below are few nuggets of knowledge concerning diet and health that I have gained throughout this journey. May it bless your life as richly as my grandfather's example has inspired mine.

SUGAR, FATS AND HEALTHY FOODS[1]

Before I made a change in my diet, I thought my eating habits were fine. I loved my pasta and white rice dishes, but I ate very little deep fried foods. I loved seafood, particularly crab and shrimp, but I tried to maintain a low-fat diet. Yes, bread and baked desserts were my weaknesses and my vegetable of choice was an iceberg lettuce salad, however, I still thought that, overall, my diet was not bad. (Oh, don't let me forget my sauces and dressings—I kind of drenched all of my foods with them. I'm talking about the ketchup, salad dressing, jelly, syrup, etc. You get the point.) Well, when I began to examine my diet, the following is the startling news that I discovered. (Yikes!) This information is broken down into the three key areas that I changed drastically after determining how much harm I was doing my body with regard to them: my intake of sugar, my understanding and choice of fats/oils, and my approach to selecting foods.

SUGAR

Medical experts suggest that simple sugar (i.e., table sugar) is the culprit of most degenerative diseases including diabetes, heart disease, arthritis, osteoporosis, kidney disease, liver disease, obesity, depression, Crohn's Disease, cancer and immune deficiency diseases such as lupus. Because cancer loves sugar, sugar is important in the growth of cancerous tumors.

Almost all sugar on the market is highly refined, and, thus all the nutrients of the molasses of the sugar cane plant that God intended for us to enjoy have been stripped away. High fructose corn syrup, an inexpensive and popular form of refined sugar, was introduced in the 1970s as a preservative for many of our processed foods and drinks. Today, this hydrolyzed fructose product can be found in many of our breads, crackers, baked goods, salad dressings, ketchup, pancake syrup, medications, and soft drinks. In fact, researchers find that the rise in obesity rates in our country correlates surprisingly well with the introduction of this product.

The danger of sugar is in its ability to depress the immune system. Research suggests that every tablespoon of sugar depresses your immune system for up to 6 hours. Consequently, some argue that if you find yourself constantly sick, sugar may be the cause.

Sugar also encourages *candida albicans overgrowth*, a yeast and a fungus that contributes to many troubling problems including female yeast infections, chronic fatigue, irritable bowel syndrome, gas and bloating, and asthma.

The current sugar substitutes that are on the market — splenda, nutrasweet, aspartame, saccharin—are arguably as bad on the body as sugar. Why? They are *artificial* sweeteners and, thus, were not made by God for our bodies to naturally digest and absorb. As Marcelle Pick, OB/GYN, NP aptly puts it (www.womentowomen.com), "Artificial sweeteners are chemicals, not food! They have no calories because they don't nourish your body in anyway — they're toxins your body has to clear, or, depending on how well you detoxify, store."

Natural sweeteners are the "natural" alternatives (no pun intended). Some of the most popular natural sweeteners are xylitol and stevia, and they can be used as direct substitutes for sugar in any dishes or drinks. The benefit of using these natural sweeteners as alternatives is that they do not trigger an insulin reaction (which, in turn, depresses the immune

system).   Xylitol is also known to have anti-cavity properties— Can you believe it? A sweetener that is actually good
for your teeth. With respect to honey, it has a similar effect
on the immune system as sugar, and so you should use it
sparingly.

Thus, beware of foods and drinks with labels that say
"low-fat," "low-calorie" and "no sugar." Generally, if you
read the labels carefully, you will find that "low-fat" means
that the fat content has been replaced with refined sugar, and
"low-calorie" and "no sugar" means that the sugar has been
replaced with artificial sweeteners.

FATS

The Atkins Diet is a very interesting diet because it suggests that you can eat all of the fat that you want as long as
you restrict your carbohydrates (sugar), which includes fruit
consumption. The problem is that all fat is not good for us
and fruit can't be bad for us—God expressly designed them
for our diet. What I have determined, though, is that some
fats are essential for our bodies to function properly, and we
place our health in jeopardy when we do not include them in
our diet.

Essential fatty acids (EFAs), known as Omega-3 and
Omega-6 fats, are the "good" fats that are necessary to
support our cardiovascular, reproductive, immune, and
nervous systems. Because they cannot be synthesized by

humans, they must be obtained in our diets. In our country, the most common EFA deficiency is the Omega-3 deficiency. Omega-3 fats can be found in nuts, flaxseed, hempseed, salmon, tuna, anchovies, sardines, wheat germ oil, canola oil (cold-pressed and unrefined), and dark leafy vegetables such as kale, collards, mustard greens, and spinach.

Omega-3 deficiency in our diets is linked to diseases such as heart disease, cancer, insulin resistance, asthma, lupus, schizophrenia, depression, accelerated aging, stroke, obesity, diabetes, arthritis, ADHD, and Alzheimer's Disease, among others.

Many folks take fish oil and flaxseed oil supplements to fulfill their Omega-3 needs. You can buy them in liquid form or pill form. (I personally prefer the liquid form.) However, if you purchase the liquid form, make sure that you buy the "cold-pressed and unrefined" kind. This simply means that the oil has not been altered from its natural (Godly) state. Also, you *must* refrigerate these liquid oils once opening. Otherwise, these oils will become rancid and potentially poisonous. My entire family takes fish oil daily (including our two boys). Now, Kevin and I have always considered Julien and Justen to be bright, however, since we have added fish oil to their diet, we have seen tremendous growth in their maturity and intellectual abilities.

For cooking purposes, extra-virgin coconut oil, extra-virgin olive oil, and canola oil are considered the healthiest of cooking oils. While extra-virgin coconut oil is a saturated fat (which most literature considers a no-no), it is the healthiest of the saturated fats. It is known to assist in weight loss (it keeps you regular), fight off infections, and support healthy thyroid functions. It also adds a subtle sweet taste to your food, to boot. While most folks are more familiar with extra-virgin olive oil, this oil can become carcinogenic at high temperatures, and, thus, is recommended mostly for sautéing foods.

At home, I try not to use hydrogenated oils of any sort (i.e., vegetable shortening, margarine, etc.). The term, "hydrogenated," similar to the terms "refined" and "hydrolyzed," means that the product has been altered from its natural (Godly) state. Furthermore, the term "hydrogenated" suggests that the process in which the product was altered added unhealthy trans fats. These fats are known to be the number one culprit of heart disease. Stay away from them!

FOODS

In preparing meals for my family nowadays, I try to keep in mind, the following suggested things:

1) **Select foods that have been maintained as close as possible to their natural state.** Look for descriptive phrases on food labels like "or-

ganic," "free-range," "minimally processed," and "whole" grains/foods. ("Free range" is a descriptive term for meat products that means that the animals have been raised in an environment where no antibiotics, hormones, and pesticides have been added.) Try to stay away from food products that have on their labels "hydrogenated," "refined," "bleached," and "hydrolyzed." Further, try to stay away from packaged meats that have been preserved in nitrites or nitrates. They have been known to cause cancer— Hormel makes some packaged lunch meats without these preservatives.

2) **Eat meals that are colorful to the eye.** Generally, that means to try to include rich-colored vegetables and fruits such as spinach, kale, broccoli greens, carrots, purple grapes, blueberries, raspberries, strawberries, apples, and oranges to your meals. These foods are densely packed with nutrients and have significant cancer-fighting properties. We have replaced white rice and bread with brown rice and whole grain bread. (They are only white because they have been bleached of all of their nutritional benefits.)

3) **Snack naturally.** Try to snacks with fruits, nuts and healthier alternatives (desserts with evaporated cane juice or alternative natural sweeteners).

4) **Be careful not to overcook foods.** Raw, mixed green salads are great vegetable dishes. When cooking vegetables, consider sautéing or grilling them to make certain that you do not cook all of the nutrients and vitamins out of them.

As far as meat choices are concerned, our family now tends to stick with chicken, turkey and fish (with scales). We have finally let go of the pork and the bottom-dwellers of the sea—crab, shrimp, lobster, scallops, clams, and catfish. (Now, that was tough!) Dr. Rex Russell, a medical doctor, has a wonderful book entitled, "What The Bible Says About Healthy Living,"[2] that really assisted us in these choices. We drink plenty of water and fresh juices, and we are big on juicing our vegetables— particularly carrots. (You have not tasted juice until you have partaken of juiced carrots and apples flavored with a hint of ginger.) Finally, I personally have added to my daily diet, wheatgrass juice and Cellfood (discussed in chapter 8) for their detoxifying and anti-cancer properties.

Here's to kicking at 100. If I don't get there, at least you will know that I tried.

CHAPTER 11

*"Thus, the heavens and the earth were finished, and all the host
of them. And on the seventh day God ended his work which he had
made; and he rested on the seventh day from all his work which he
had made. And God blessed the seventh day, and sanctified it;
because that in it he had rested from all his work which God created
and made." Genesis 2: 1-3*

There is no restoration without "rest."

From: Cynthia
Sent: Wed 04/18/2007 11:23 AM
To: Prayer Sisters
Subject: 4.18 Update/Prayer

Sisters,

First, I would like to thank God for blessing me to be formally completed with all my standard care and treatments. I will not need to go back to see my doctor again until another 3 mos. Now, I am in just the process of recovery. Some hair is growing back~ I've got a little fuzz on the top now. I am still looking forward to the eyebrows growing back~ I've come to learn that drawing in eyebrows is an art form (*smile*).   Since my last email, I did lose some eyelashes as well, but fortunately they did not all leave me. I am still a bit anemic, but otherwise, I feel good. What I've learned from this part of my journey is more than I can write in this email, but I will share with you at a later time...

-Cynthia

From: Cynthia
Sent: Mon 05/14/2007 9:53 AM
To: Prayer Sisters
Subject: 5/14/07 Update

Hello Sisters,

I pray that all of my sister-moms had a beautiful Mother's Day. Just wanted to give you a brief update. Y'all, I am doing well! I mentioned to you in a previous email that I lost my eyebrows and quite a few of my eyelashes. Would you believe, though, that within two and a half weeks, they had returned. Praise God! The hair is growing back. Still not thick enough to do anything with it, but it is filling in a bit more everyday. Now, the funny part is that my hair is currently growing back in bone straight, not an African wave or curl in sight!!! (LOL) In my prayer time here recently, I told the Lord to hurry up and stop playing with me and let me see what my real hair is gonna look like before I start telling y'all about my Indian side of the family (HA!!~ I do, though, really have some Indian in my family, don't I mom?)

Also, the energy level is getting so much better that I have decided to participate in my first Susan G. Komen 5K Race for the Cure on June 2, 2007 as a cancer survivor (hey, hey, hey!). I will be participating in the race in Washington, DC along with my baby sister, Frances, on a team aptly named, "Sisters Walking In Victory (SWV)." While this year I plan to walk, next year, it is my goal to be running for the Lord!

Lastly, I want you to go ahead and pencil in my post-praise party date for Saturday, January 5, 2008, exactly one year from my pre-praise party. Planning committee, get ready! What a victorious time we're going to have! Until next time...

Love ya,
Cynthia

When I had my sons, I quickly gained a whole new appreciation for my mother, Mary P. Williams. As I struggled with balancing my new responsibilities of being a mother with those of being a wife and career woman, I was at a loss for how my mom did this with *four* children. She was a middle school teacher during the day, taxied us children back and forth to different activities in the afternoons, cooked dinner *every* evening, and made sure that we all were bathed and in the bed by 8pm each night.

I had only two boys, but could barely prepare meals daily (notice I said "prepare"—there is a difference), and on any given night, you could call my house and hear one of them in the background still up as late as 11pm at night. I was always tired and stressed, and constantly on the move as I attempted to accomplish all that I "must" do. My poor husband was always complaining about not having enough "us" time, but I could not figure out how to fit everything in the twenty-four hours of the day. My mom used to tell me all the time that I needed to slow down, but I could not imagine how this could happen with all of the things on my to-do list that were still incomplete. Ripping and running, that's all I knew how to do, until…I got sick.

Boy, what a mental paradigm shift that was. Overnight, I went from being in constant motion to coming to a complete halt. Moreover, as I stood still for probably the first time in twenty years, I realized that most of my "busy-ness" was by *choice*. Most of my deadlines were self-imposed. Most of my "have-to-dos" were really "want-to-dos." Most of my "right nows" were really "can waits." Wow.

And so, I found myself at a crossroads. I had to make a decision. Was I going to continue to try to iron out every detail of my life, or hang-dry and enjoy the wrinkles?

I have decided the latter. I would rather be wrinkled and here than to be perfectly laid out. Ha!

CONCLUSION: AND YOU KNOW
WHAT ELSE?

CHAPTER 12

"Now unto Him that is able to do exceeding abundantly above all that we ask or think, according to the power that worketh in us, unto Him be glory in the church by Christ Jesus throughout all ages, world without end. Amen." (Ephesians 3:20,21)

Exceedingly gracious He is. Exceedingly grateful I am.

From: Cynthia
Sent: Thu 05/31/2007 10:47 AM
To: Prayer Sisters
Subject: 5/31/07 Update

Good Morning Sisters,

As I shared with many of you during my pre-praise party in January, one of the first times the Lord spoke into my spirit concerning my certain victory over breast cancer occurred shortly after my husband's aunt, Aunt Edith, shared with me about her sister-in-law's diagnosis of breast cancer over forty-four years ago. This was days after I had first learned in October that I had breast cancer. My Aunt Edith had called with words of encouragement indicating that her sister-in-law was still strutting (*smile*), and that she could always keep up with how long she had been a survivor because she had been pregnant with her twins, Debbie and Donna, when her sister-in-law was diagnosed. At that time, Aunt Edith's words were so comforting because that was the longest time I had personally heard of someone beating cancer. Doctors had talked about 5, 10, and 15 year survivorship, but I wanted to hear stories of people who had survived 40 and 50+ years, so Aunt Edith's phone call was so uplifting.

But while I thought God's sole reason for having Aunt Edith share with me this at that time was to encourage me, God was setting the stage for something even more unreal. My sister, Celia, and her husband had been trying for several years to have kids (and we all know how that is). Anyhow, as we sat in the waiting room this past November waiting for me to be called back for my first surgery, Celia shares with me that she was expecting. Praise God, right?!! Well, not only was she expecting one child, but two~ TWINS!! Come on, y'all~ how clearly can God speak! It was as if God was saying to me, "Just like your aunt has kept up with her sister-in-law's victory by the age of her twins, so shall your sister keep up with your victory report (by the age of her twins)." HALLELUJAH!! I shared with my sister right there in the waiting room what God placed in my spirit. It was confirmation for her too because of her prior difficult experiences and she wasn't sure how successful her pregnancy would be. We cried, claiming victory that morning for both of us.........I'm sorry, I must pause........God is SO good! And this is what I held onto going into my first surgery and throughout my treatments.

Well, I said all of this to say, "Guess where I'm going this weekend?" To my sister's twin baby shower! This weekend God is bringing full circle what He promised in my spirit the morning of November 20th. Celia is due in early July with twin boys. And this is JUST the beginning of God's fulfillment of His promise regarding this event in my life. Stay tuned.

On another note, women, the scarves and wigs are now off. God has been faithful in allowing me to have enough hair to go natural during this hot summer (God really knows how much we can bear~ wigs are just TOO hot for me!) So now, when you see me, I will be stepping with my ultra low hairdo. My official unveiling (LOL) will fittingly take place this weekend when I take my victory stroll down the streets of Washington, D.C. for the Susan Komen 5k Run/Walk Saturday morning and then serve as host for my sister's baby shower that afternoon in Maryland. (Many thanks to those of you who provided support for my 5k walk!)

I've still got more to tell, so until next time, just know that my story is because of His glory......

Prayerfully indebted to you,
Cynthia

From: Cynthia
Sent: Mon 06/25/2007 9:48 AM
To: Prayer Sisters
Subject: 6/25/07 Update

Good Morning Sisters,

God is good (ALWAYS)! My sister had her twin boys, Lawson Taylor (5 lbs., 14 oz; 20 in.) and Bryson Eli (5 lbs., 13 oz.; 19 in.), this past Friday, June 22, 2007. Of course, our family is ecstatic! Again, God is honoring what He said way back in November. I am doing fantastic. A couple of weeks ago, I power-walked in the Susan Komen 5K Run/Walk with 45,000 others (WOW) in DC. It was an amazing experience. I unveiled my new hairdo there, and have been strutting ever since (*smile*)...

-Cynthia

From: Cynthia
Sent: Wed 10/3/2007 5:15 PM
To: Prayer Sisters
Subject: 10.03.07 Update

Hey Sistergirlfriends,

I know. I know. I haven't corresponded in a looong time. I've gotten a few emails and phone calls lately checking up on me. Thank you so much for the luv! I am doing well, girls. Tired, but well. I am going to make this short because I will give you a full update after the women's conference this weekend and my 6-month check-up on Tuesday, Oct. 9. Please keep me in your prayers that God uses me in a mighty way this weekend as well as allows me to be a witness in the doctor's office on Tuesday. Talk at ya on the other side. Luv ya!

-Cynthia

From: Cynthia
Sent: Wed 10/10/2007 12:35 AM
To: Prayer Sisters
Subject: 10.10.07 Update

Sisters,

Where do I begin? Talk about a weekend of support, encouragement, and empowerment (SEE)! As I shared earlier, I was in Va. Beach participating in SEE Ministries "Yes, You Can Girl" Conference (www.seeministries.com) this past weekend. It was SO blessed. Thank you SO much for your prayers. You just don't know how your prayers served as a conduit this weekend directly from Heaven to me. Further, I was so encouraged by the seasoned and sage women of God who presented, shared and kept it REAL!

As for my 6-month check-up~ Well, my mammogram came back negative (hey, hey!). My red blood cell count is at higher levels than it was before I began the healing process, and, thus, my anemia is gone (hey, hey, hey!). All of my vitals are good. In fact, I was also due for my annual physical which is the first since my change in diet and lifestyle. And can I testify? My LDL cholesterol level went from 152 last year to 110 this year. My doctor literally asked, "What the heck did you do?!" Some of you may have thought I may have went a bit on the deep end with my diet changes (with my fish oil~, freshly juiced vegetables~, wheatgrass juice~, flax oil/cottage cheese/blueberry mix~, cellfood~, organic and all-wheat~, no refined~, no enriched~ diet). But prayer alone did not change my cholesterol level and my current physical health, particularly when my doctor just a year ago wanted to chalk my high cholesterol up to my genetics and wanted to put me on medication. You can't tell me that there is not something to when you follow God's diet. Y'all God is just so good!

-Cynthia

P.S. By the way, I forgot to mention one thing...My oncologist said to me something very interesting when she was looking at my vitals Tuesday. She said, "Keep doing what you are doing because at the rate you are going, you will live forever." Y'all know I had to jump on top of that, didn't you?! I replied, "Doctor J, you have now gone spiritual on me. I KNOW I am going to live forever!"

To God be the glory! Amen.

NOTES

Chapter 4

1. Name has been changed.

Chapter 7

1. Thank you, Mrs. Diann Beard, for blessing me with such an invaluable resource over twenty years ago. Who would have thought that it would be needed for such a time as this.

2. Ron Rhodes, *The Complete Book of Bible Promises* (Eugene, OR: Harvest House, 2003).

Chapter 10

1. Taken from various sources, including:

   http://trusted.md/blog/vreni_gurd/2007/02/15/ sugar_the_disease_generator

   http://www.womentowomen.com/ nutritionandweightloss/splenda.aspx

   http://goodfats.pamrotella.com

   http://www.risingstarlc.com/coconut.pdf

http://www.biblicalhealthinstitute.com

http://www.luminahealth.com/products/
cellfood.htm

2. Rex Russell, M.D., *What the Bible Says About Healthy Living* (Grand Rapids, MI: Revell, 1999).

NOTES

Chapter 4

1. Name has been changed.

Chapter 7

1. Thank you, Mrs. Diann Beard, for blessing me with such an invaluable resource over twenty years ago. Who would have thought that it would be needed for such a time as this.

2. Ron Rhodes, *The Complete Book of Bible Promises* (Eugene, OR: Harvest House, 2003).

Chapter 10

1. Taken from various sources, including:

   http://trusted.md/blog/vreni_gurd/2007/02/15/sugar_the_disease_generator

   http://www.womentowomen.com/nutritionandweightloss/splenda.aspx

   http://goodfats.pamrotella.com

   http://www.risingstarlc.com/coconut.pdf

http://www.biblicalhealthinstitute.com

http://www.luminahealth.com/products/
cellfood.htm

2. Rex Russell, M.D., *What the Bible Says About Healthy Living* (Grand Rapids, MI: Revell, 1999).